Praise for *Are You Tired and W*

"*So many of us are addicted to a fast-paced, hectic life supported by coffee, sugar, and adrenaline. Unfortunately this is a prescription for burnout and disease, but thankfully, in* **Are You Tired and Wired?**, *Marcelle Pick explains why our sleep-deprived, over-caffeinated, stress-driven habits are depleting us and provides a practical, step-by-step plan for finding our pause buttons and restoring our health and vitality. If you are exhausted, drained, and heading toward burnout, read this book, and save yourself.*"

— **Mark Hyman, M.D.**, *New York Times* best-selling author
of *The UltraMind Solution* and *UltraMetabolism*

"*Marcelle Pick has written a book that is relevant, personal, and provides practical solutions to recognizing and understanding adrenal fatigue. Her descriptions will resonate with those who are wired and tired. It's a great validation to understand what's happening to you. This book blends the best of the scientific and clinical to provide a personal guide with specific action steps to help you find the road to recovery.*"

— **Liz Lipski, Ph.D., CCN**, author of *Digestive Wellness* and *Digestive Wellness for Children*, Director of Doctoral Studies, Hawthorn University

"*Marcelle Pick continues to be at the leading edge of women's health care by listening to her patients and responding to their pain.* **Are You Tired and Wired?** *is exactly what the many women suffering from undiagnosed adrenal fatigue need. I'll be recommending it to my patients.*"

— **Frank Lipman, M.D.**, author of *Spent* and *Total Renewal*

"*Marcelle Pick is a compassionate and insightful clinician who has taken her understanding of healing to a new level. Her synthesis of the functional medicine/systems-biology approach gives practical hands-on tools for patients to apply in their lives. I have worked with these tools in practice and find them to be invaluable in the nearly 40 percent of patients I see, across all medical conditions, who are 'tired and wired.'*"

— **Patrick J. Hanaway, M.D.**, President, American Board
of Integrative Holistic Medicine

"From working with thousands of patients, Marcelle understands the crucial linkage between stress and illness and she also knows what to do about it. She gives each of us the power to heal ourselves. While based on impeccable research and science, her recommendations are surprisingly easy to follow. Marcelle is a healer and through her work you'll discover that you are too."

— **Raz Ingrasci**, President and CEO, Hoffman Institute Foundation

"Marcelle's new book is amazing. She has taken complicated hormonal processes and made them simple for everyone to understand. I love her list of 'adrenal-friendly activities.' They are quick, easy, and portable. The many case studies illustrate that adrenal stress and fatigue comes in a broad number of varieties. Most women will see themselves—and be inspired to take action to restore their adrenals . . . and their life. Thank you for this much-needed book."

— **Dr. Sherri Tenpenny**, President, Tenpenny Integrative Medical Center and author of *Saying No to Vaccines*

Are You Tired and Wired?

ALSO BY MARCELLE PICK

Book

THE CORE BALANCE DIET: 4 Weeks to Boost
Your Metabolism and Lose Weight for Good

CD

CORE BALANCE: Boost Your Metabolism
and Lose Weight for Good

All of the above are available at your local
bookstore, or may be ordered by visiting:

Hay House USA: **www.hayhouse.com**®
Hay House Australia: **www.hayhouse.com.au**
Hay House UK: **www.hayhouse.co.uk**
Hay House South Africa: **www.hayhouse.co.za**
Hay House India: **www.hayhouse.co.in**

Are You Tired and Wired?

Your Proven 30-Day Program for Overcoming Adrenal Fatigue and Feeling Fantastic Again

MARCELLE PICK

MSN, OB/GYN NP, co-founder of Women to Women

HAY HOUSE, INC.
Carlsbad, California • New York City
London • Sydney • Johannesburg
Vancouver • Hong Kong • New Delhi

Published and distributed in the United States by: Hay House, Inc.: www.hayhouse.com •
Published and distributed in Australia by: Hay House Australia Pty. Ltd.: www.hayhouse.com.au
• *Published and distributed in the United Kingdom by:* Hay House UK, Ltd.: www.hayhouse.co.uk
• *Published and distributed in the Republic of South Africa by:* Hay House SA (Pty), Ltd.:
www.hayhouse.co.za • *Distributed in Canada by:* Raincoast: www.raincoast.com • *Published in
India by:* Hay House Publishers India: www.hayhouse.co.in

Design: Tricia Breidenthal
Indexer: Jay Kreider

Library of Congress Cataloging-in-Publication Data

Pick, Marcelle
 Are you tired and wired? : your proven 30-day program for overcoming adrenal fatigue and feeling
fantastic again / Marcelle Pick. -- 1st ed.
      p. cm.
 Includes bibliographical references and index.
 ISBN 978-1-4019-2819-3 (hardcover : alk. paper) 1. Adrenal glands--Diseases. 2. Fatigue. 3. Stress
(Physiology) I. Title.
 RC659.P53 2011
 616.4'5--dc22

                                2010047505

Tradepaper ISBN: 978-1-4019-2820-9
Digital ISBN: 978-1-4019-3088-2

15 14 13 12   6 5 4 3
1st edition, March 2011
3rd edition, August 2012

Printed in the United States of America

*I'm dedicating this book to my children,
who have been the ones to teach me the
importance of balance and who have called me
to task when I was out of balance. Without
their support and inspiration, this book
would never have been written.*

*I also dedicate this book to my patients,
in the hopes that every woman will have a
life that works for her, because we're all
always trying to do so much, so well.*

CONTENTS

INTRODUCTION:

A New Diagnosis

- Do you feel exhausted, overwhelmed, and stressed all the time?

- Do you need five cups of coffee or a constant infusion of soda just to make it through the day?

- Do you have trouble waking up, falling asleep, or staying asleep, no matter which herbal supplements you try?

- Do you find yourself feeling constantly irritable or on edge?

- Do you feel that you need to exercise to stay in shape even though you're exhausted when you do?

- Do you feel as though everything you eat turns to fat?

- Are you always hungry, frequently craving sweets, or tempted by "carbo-binges"?

- Are you plagued by irregular or painful periods or PMS?

- Are you struggling with perimenopause or menopause: lowered sex drive, vaginal dryness, mood swings, and hot flashes?

- Do you find yourself feeling forgetful, "foggy," or unable to concentrate?

- Do you find that you do better when you're always on the go?

- Do you find that you actually enjoy adrenaline rushes and feel a little bored without a crisis to handle?

- Are you struggling with anxiety, depression, or despair?

Sound familiar? If I've painted a picture you recognize—in yourself, in your family, among your friends and colleagues—you've just gotten a good look at *adrenal dysfunction,* a distressingly common problem in which overworked adrenal glands combined with lifelong emotional patterns add up to a painful set of physical, mental, and emotional symptoms. In the early stages of adrenal dysfunction, you might feel "tired and wired": keyed up, anxious, fatigued, and depressed. In the later stages, you might simply feel exhausted. Either way, you know something's wrong—even if your health-care provider has assured you that you're fine or hasn't included adrenal dysfunction in his or her diagnosis.

You may not think much about your adrenals, but they are crucial to your health, mood, and well-being. These little triangular-shaped glands sit on top of the kidneys, responsible for giving us those extra surges of vitality that we need to cope with unusual challenges, new demands, and heightened levels of stress. That vitality is commonly known as the fight-or-flight reaction. When a major challenge threatens, our adrenal glands kick up the stress hormones, enabling us to cope with whatever challenge or emergency befalls. Then, when the crisis is over, the stress hormones subside and we relax once more.

But our adrenals don't just operate during emergencies; they're on duty all day long. Under ordinary circumstances, our adrenals are designed to give us relatively small blasts of strength, from the little burst of energy that wakes us up in the morning to the stimulating hormones that keep us awake, alert, and focused throughout the day. Ideally, as evening comes, our adrenal production is supposed to steadily decline, allowing us to relax into a restful sleep.

That's how our adrenals were meant to work. But when we're chronically under stress, our adrenals are forced to behave very differently. Instead of just enough stress hormones to keep us alert and awake, with occasional extras for a fight-or-flight emergency, our adrenals are being asked to provide stress hormones for a continual barrage of challenges as they help us cope with the latest crisis from the kids or meeting that new deadline at work—and then drag ourselves out of bed a few hours later to start all over again.

Our stress may come from life events: challenges at home or at work. Or perhaps our stress comes from environmental toxins that place an undue burden on our bodies; or from noisy, unpleasant surroundings; or from chronic infection, asthma, allergies, or pain. We may be acting out the effects of *historical stress:* reactions to present-day events that are made more difficult or intense because of our past experiences, especially those involving our parents. Maybe we're facing a difficult combination of life events, health problems, *and* environmental stressors. However it happens, too many of us are living in a condition of near-constant stress, with no true downtime for our bodies, minds, and spirits. Adrenal dysfunction is the result.

Unfortunately, your health-care practitioner is likely to ignore or dismiss adrenals as the source of your problem unless you are suffering from either Addison's disease, in which your adrenals severely underproduce, or Cushing's syndrome, in which they severely overproduce. These two conditions are well understood by conventional medicine—thank heavens! But if your adrenal imbalance is less extreme—as is true for hundreds of thousands of U.S. women—your practitioner is unlikely to recognize your condition. That's because, despite the enormous body of science relating adrenal problems to a wide variety of symptoms, adrenal dysfunction is not a commonly accepted diagnosis.

The good news is that once you *have* identified adrenal dysfunction as your condition, you can address all your symptoms and heal the underlying problem that is causing them. You can change your diet, adjust your lifestyle, and reprogram the emotional patterns that are stressing you out—and you can do it in 30 days. Within a month, you'll see a significant difference. Within two months, you'll find that many of your symptoms have disappeared. And within three months or more, you'll have made a great beginning toward restoring your adrenal balance, restarting your metabolism, and regaining your natural energy.

That's what happened with my patient Tanya. An attractive woman in her late 30s with a sweet, friendly smile, Tanya seemed energized and "up" as she introduced herself to me and thanked me for seeing her. But as soon as she had made that initial effort, I could tell that she was completely exhausted.

"I don't know what's wrong with me," she confessed. "I just don't feel at all like myself. I used to be able to finish a day at work and then go out to a movie or a club. But now I'm so wiped out I can barely drag myself home. I fall into bed exhausted—but then I wake up in the middle of the night and can't get back to sleep. My periods are really irregular and I'm having lots of cramps, which is just not me. And even though I'm really, *really* good about sticking to my diet, somehow I've put on ten pounds in the last three months, and no matter what I do, I just can't seem to shake it."

Tanya looked at me, her large hazel eyes suddenly brimming with tears. "I've been to two different doctors," she continued. "One said there's nothing really wrong with me and I should just decrease my stress, get some more sleep on the weekends, and maybe do some yoga. But I've tried all that, and it doesn't make any difference. He wanted to put me on antidepressants—but is that really what I need? The other guy said

I should cut back on high-fat foods and be more disciplined about exercising, but I'm down to 1,200 calories a day as it is, and sometimes I'm just too tired to exercise, I really am. I'm at the end of my rope."

I looked at Tanya, still trying valiantly to control her tears, and I thought about the thousands of other patients who had sat in that chair, telling me similar stories. Once it was LeAnn, a 35-year-old marketing executive and mother of two, who had mysteriously gained 20 pounds over the past year and whose once-abundant black hair had started to thin. Another time it was Emily, a 52-year-old professor of art history with a high school–age son and a daughter in college, who had become so exhausted that she needed a morning nap and an afternoon nap just to make it through the day. Then there was Christa, the perky 28-year-old film editor who had come to me because of her out-of-control PMS symptoms and the constant infusion of soy lattes and diet sodas that she needed to get her through the day.

On the surface, these women seemed very different. But all of them were suffering from adrenal dysfunction—and no wonder. They had each been driving themselves to the point where their bodies just couldn't take it anymore. Their adrenal systems had been asked to respond once too often to a last-minute deadline; a weekly round of chauffeuring the kids; or nonstop months of work, social, and personal obligations; and they didn't understand how important it was to take some downtime every day. Now either their adrenals were flooding their systems with excessive levels of stress hormones, causing them to feel both tired and wired, or else their adrenal reserves were dwindling, creating a virtually constant state of exhaustion.

I tested Tanya, as I test all of my patients, to rule out other potential causes for her condition, such as Addison's disease and Cushing's syndrome. I also gave her the tests that I and other functional-medicine practitioners use to determine more subtle forms of adrenal dysfunction. (Functional medicine is a science-based approach to healing that adopts an individualized approach to each patient, with a focus on prevention and on addressing a condition's underlying causes.) For Tanya, LeAnn, Emily, and Christa, their test results and their symptoms were all saying the same thing: their adrenals were seriously out of balance.

How Your Biography Becomes Your Biology

I've borrowed this phrase from healer and best-selling author Caroline Myss because I think it sums up so beautifully the other key factor behind adrenal dysfunction. No matter how disciplined we are about cleaning up our diet, taking our nutritional supplements, and getting regular exercise, if we don't attend to the emotional piece of the puzzle, our adrenal symptoms won't go away.

Here are some of the questions I ask my patients as we work through their biography-biology connection:

- Do you worry about not being good enough, not doing enough, never really finishing anything, not accomplishing all you set out to do, not working at the level you expect from yourself?

- Do you push yourself constantly, no matter what?

- Do you find yourself frequently worried about what people think about you and spend a lot of emotional energy on getting them to see you in a good light?

- Do you spend more time thinking about other people's needs than your own?

- Do you find yourself saying at the end of each day that you forgot to exercise because you were so busy taking care of everybody else?

- Do you frequently work that extra hour (or four!) to get everything "just right" and then arrive home exhausted because every day gets longer?

- Do you often berate yourself about what you have done and how you have done it, especially if you made mistakes?

- Do you feel you must do everything perfectly?

- Do you believe you must keep all your emotions buried deep inside?

- Do you believe that you can never be vulnerable and show your true frailty?

- Do you tell yourself on a regular basis how fat or stupid you are?

- Do you find yourself experiencing the same frustrating or disappointing situations over and over again?

You've just gotten a look at the emotional component of being tired and wired, the compulsion that so many of us feel to meet other people's needs, expectations, or demands at our own expense. This emotional component doesn't just remain "in your mind" or "in your feelings." Feeling stressed triggers an actual physical response, a complex cascade of hormones and neurotransmitters whose side effects include weight gain, blood-sugar dysregulation, menstrual problems, thyroid abnormalities, digestive problems, hormone imbalances, immune and autoimmune conditions, cardiovascular issues, and exhaustion. Those hormones also affect your brain, creating memory problems, the inability to concentrate, irritability, anxiety, and depression.

Why do we feel stressed in the first place? We might be responding to a real-life situation, our boss yelling at us, for example, or our partner showing up three hours late for dinner. But we might also be responding to *historical stress:* the emotional echoes from our past. Whenever our boss speaks sharply to us, it might trigger the childhood panic we felt whenever our father began to yell. If our partner shows up late for a meal, it might evoke our childhood sorrow that our mother was often absent. Our adrenals are working overtime not only because of present stress (our boss's tone and our partner's lateness may not be such a big deal), but also because of stress from the past (our father's anger and our mother's absence were very painful and upsetting). Driven by our biographies as well as by our current circumstances, our bodies go into stress mode far more often—and more intensely—than they need to. Adrenal dysfunction is the result.

Adrenal Dysfunction: Diagnosis of the Future?

In my opinion, adrenal dysfunction will be a completely accepted diagnosis within about 25 years or so, and it will then be "standard of care" for physicians and practitioners of all types to properly test for it and treat it. The science to support this notion—in such prestigious publications as *The New England Journal of Medicine, Psychoneuroimmunology,* and *Neuroscience & Biobehavioral Reviews*—has been well documented. But as we've seen with many other conditions, standard medical practice often takes time to catch up with cutting-edge research. (If you're interested in knowing more about the scientific work on which I relied to write this book, check out the Further Reading references in the endnotes of this book or take a look at the bibliographic section of my website, www.MarcellePick.com.)

Intellectually, I understand how busy practitioners are and how overwhelmed they can become at the prospect of keeping up with the plethora of new scientific studies that seem to get more numerous every year. But emotionally, I find it frustrating that so many of my colleagues still argue with me—not over how to treat adrenal dysfunction, but over whether the condition even exists. Those of us who work in functional medicine know of tests that can capture adrenal dysfunction and of treatments that can heal it. There's simply no good reason for this condition not to be recognized and treated.

Studies have shown, though, that it takes standard medical practice at least 50 years to catch up with research—and we've had the data on adrenal dysfunction for just about 25 years. Here's hoping that 25 years from now, this book will be completely irrelevant—because you've learned everything in these pages from your own medical practitioner!

Take Action to Feel Better

This book is your resource. I'll help you identify some of the emotional stressors that have been contributing to lifelong patterns of behavior—patterns that continue to create tremendous emotional and physical stress. I'll also identify an adrenal-friendly program of diet, nutritional supplements, and lifestyle changes individually tailored to your adrenal type. And I'll help you reprogram both your emotions and your body so that you can stop being tired and wired and start feeling like yourself again. To me, this is truly empowering, because knowing our biography often means that we can change our biology.

As you read this book, look to Part I for a complete explanation of what's going on with your body—and for all the emotional components that so frequently accompany this debilitating condition. Then turn to Part II for a step-by-step guide to feeling terrific sooner than you'd think possible—and how to create a life that will continue to support your health.

I've seen thousands of patients get better with this approach, and you can, too. So let's get started. All the help you need is right here.

PART I

Why Are You Tired and Wired?

Every day, I see patients who are suffering from adrenal dysfunction, tired and wired women who all too often have been to practitioners who dismiss their symptoms as "not enough willpower," "stressed in general," or worst of all, "just getting older." Despite cutting-edge research published in major medical journals, myths and misinformation abound.

But I'm here to tell you that adrenal dysfunction is real—and that we can do something about it. Once you understand *why* you are tired and wired, you will feel better, I promise, because you will finally have some idea of what's happening. In two decades of practice I've treated literally thousands of women struggling with this problem, and I can tell you exactly what I tell them. We can absolutely do something about this.

The first step, as always, is awareness: understanding what causes adrenal dysfunction. That's what I'll share with you in the next four chapters. I promise that you'll find this information empowering and reassuring, an important first step in becoming friends with your body.

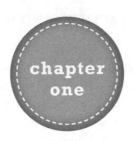
RECOGNIZING ADRENAL DYSFUNCTION

Marcy is a 27-year-old emergency-room nurse. She's on her feet all day, responding to the intense demands of her patients, their families, the doctors, and often, the hospital administrators as well. When Marcy started her job, she had boundless energy, but lately she's been slowing down a little, passing up nights with "the girls" to zone out in front of the TV. She's always been a little careless about her diet, and her exercise habits are irregular at best. Still, for most of her life, she has remained close to her ideal weight—until now, when she's begun to put on a few pounds. Marcy has a boyfriend whom she likes a lot, but she's noticed that lately, her sex drive isn't what it used to be. None of these concerns are significant enough to send Marcy to the doctor, but when she comes in for her regular checkup, she can't help being worried. She asks me, "Aren't I too young to feel this way?"

Lisa is a 38-year-old graphic designer who works for a medium-sized advertising agency. Her work goes in cycles: for weeks, things are relatively slow and peaceful, and then she'll have two weeks of "deadline hell," putting in 14 or even 16 hours a day as hard-to-please or stressed-out clients expect her to perform miracles. Lisa's 14-year-old daughter challenges Lisa's authority constantly, but she's also upset that her mom isn't home more and complains frequently that Lisa isn't available for more "mother-daughter stuff." Lisa's husband is a salesman who's away on business trips half the week and is cranky and exhausted the other half. When Lisa comes in for her yearly checkup, she gradually shares with me a number of problems: intense PMS symptoms, vaginal dryness, thinning hair, a slow but steady weight gain, difficulty concentrating, forgetfulness, increased irritability, and a habit of waking up at 2 A.M., her heart racing. "I'm not happy about all this," Lisa says when I ask her how she feels about this long list of issues. "But what am I supposed to do about it? My life is just out of control."

Jolene is a 52-year-old high school principal and a mother of three. She has assumed primary responsibility for her elderly mother and also for her husband's parents, all of whom live in town. Jolene has always struggled with her weight, but now it's really out of control: more than 50 pounds above her ideal. She's tried to start a mild exercise program, walking 30 minutes a day, three days a week, but most weeks she can barely manage even one session. She comes home each day exhausted but somehow manages to drag herself out at night: to a church group, a Neighborhood Watch meeting, or one of her kids' events. On the weekends she has her kids, church, her mother, and her in-laws.

Although she feels tired all the time, Jolene usually has trouble falling asleep at night, so the next day, she's even more tired. She's been suffering from hot flashes, and her bone-density readings aren't what they should be. She's also discouraged about what she perceives to be a real fraying in her family's fabric. "We're all so busy all the time, we never really talk to each other," she tells me. "Pretty soon the kids will be off at college, and I feel like Malcolm and I will have just missed everything. And as for the two of us, don't get me started! We barely talk to each other anymore, let alone anything else."

The Misunderstood Condition

Marcy, Lisa, and Jolene are each struggling with *adrenal dysfunction*, a widespread problem that affects women of all ages. Do you think you might be among them? Take a look at the following symptoms and see if they sound familiar.

Physical Symptoms

- You're tired when you wake up in the morning—even if you've supposedly gotten a good night's sleep.

- You often can't stay awake in the evenings.

- You have trouble falling asleep and/or staying asleep.

- You frequently find yourself falling asleep in the afternoon.

- You feel both wired *and* exhausted.

- If you sit down quietly in a warm spot—to read, meditate, or just to rest for a moment—you find yourself dozing off as soon as you feel the least bit relaxed.

- If you're forced to sit and wait for a few minutes—perhaps in a doctor's office or at your kids' school—you suddenly feel completely exhausted.

- If you quickly sit up or stand up, you feel light-headed or dizzy (a common sign of *hypotension,* or low blood pressure).

- You often feel dizzy, not just when you stand up.

- Your blood pressure is often low, or varies between high and low.

- You frequently struggle with diarrhea, indigestion, or other digestive problems.

- You have heart palpitations.

- You frequently feel weak all over.

- You have a tendency to gain weight around your waistline.

- You are losing muscle mass and gaining fat.

- You can't tolerate exercise the way you used to.

- You feel unwell much of the time or you often come down with a lot of "little things"—colds, flu, infections.

- You're always cold (which may also be a sign of thyroid problems).

- You have frequent headaches.

- Your ankles are swollen.

- You retain water.

- You have dark circles under your eyes.

- Your mouth is often dry.

- When you're nervous, your hands and feet sweat.

- You struggle with *hypoglycemia* (low blood sugar) and feel shaky or awful if you miss a meal.

- You frequently crave high-protein foods, salt, or sweets.

- You can't make it through the day without frequent infusions of coffee and/or regular starchy or sugary snacks.

- You are struggling with intense symptoms of PMS, perimenopause, or menopause.

Psychological Symptoms

- You're irritable and quick to lose your temper.

- You're prone to road rage or become extremely angry over little things.

- You feel as though you're constantly on edge, ready to "lose it" at the least little thing.

- You feel listless, depressed, or emotionally numb.

- Your sex drive is low.

- You frequently have nightmares.

- You often feel an overpowering urge to cry.

- You have trouble concentrating or feel mentally foggy.

- You suffer from free-floating anxiety.

- You are easily startled.

- You simply feel stressed all the time.

- Everything seems like a chore.

As you can see, some of the symptoms are contradictory: can't sleep/can't stay awake; always on edge/listless and depressed. That's because adrenal dysfunction is a progressive condition that moves through successive phases, manifesting differently as the condition gets worse. The condition also shows up differently in different women, primarily as three main types. Although the following are not hard-and-fast medical categories, they are the general patterns I have observed throughout two decades of practice. See if they apply to you or to the women you know:

Type 1, "The Racehorse": The Racehorse feels speedy and energized all day, fueled by high levels of stress hormones that keep her alert and on point. Those same excess hormones, though, produce a number of unwanted symptoms: extra weight, digestive difficulties, blood-pressure irregularities, irritability, and sex-hormone imbalances that can in turn create difficulties with premenstrual syndrome, menstrual periods, perimenopause, and menopause. Used to multitasking at top speed, the Racehorse is periodically over-whelmed with fatigue.

Type 2, "The Workhorse": Exhausted in the morning when her stress-hormone levels are low, the Workhorse has a hard time waking up. She mainlines caffeine to keep herself going, but for much of the day, she's exhausted. Then at night, stimulated by the daylong infusion of coffee, soda, or energy drinks, her stress hormones peak. Either she can't fall asleep or she can't stay asleep, waking in the wee hours to find that her mind is racing, her heart is pounding, and her anxiety refuses to go away. She too suffers from a long list of symptoms, including weight gain, decreased sex drive, thyroid problems, digestive difficulties, and sometimes depression.

Type 3, "The Flatliner": Either the Racehorse or the Workhorse might end up a Flatliner—someone whose store of adrenal reserves is simply exhausted. The Flatliner tries hard to meet the needs of her family, friends, and colleagues, but she's barely able to summon the energy to go to work or to play with her children. Despite her fatigue, she rarely enjoys a restful sleep, often waking up as tired as when she lay down. Like the other two types, she struggles with a number of medical issues as well as weight gain, decreased sex drive, and depression, and she's beginning to wonder if she'll ever feel like herself again.

Because the adrenals produce so many of the biochemicals that the body needs to function, women with adrenal problems often have trouble in a wide variety of ways: blood-sugar dysregulation; thyroid abnormalities; sex-hormone imbalances; digestive difficulties; cardiovascular problems; immune and autoimmune conditions; mood disorders such as anxiety and depression; and cognitive problems, such as poor memory, fogginess, and an inability to concentrate. It can also work the other way around: any type of physical or emotional problem tends to create more stress for our bodies, which in turn can contribute to adrenal dysfunction. This proliferation of symptoms can make adrenal dysfunction difficult to identify. But if you know what you're looking for, it can be done.

Zeroing In on a Diagnosis

If you suspect you might be struggling with adrenal dysfunction, you'll want to work with your health practitioner to rule out other conditions. Ask him or her about the following tests:

- Thyroid: TSH, free T3, free T4, and reverse T3. You may also be checked for antithyroid autoantibodies, such as thyroid peroxidase antibodies, antithyroglobulin antibodies, antimicrosomal antibodies, and thyroid-stimulating immunoglobulins, to help identify any autoimmune component. Further thyroid evaluation may include a thyroxine-binding globulin, and perhaps a TRH stimulation test. A basal body-temperature test and a thyroid-symptom questionnaire can additionally help diagnose thyroid problems.

- CMP (comprehensive metabolic profile) to look for other health problems

- Fasting glucose and insulin tests, and insulin and glucose testing conducted two hours after a high-sugar meal, which is known as a "two-hour postprandial test," to look at blood-sugar and insulin dysregulation

- Hemoglobin A1c, to evaluate blood sugars over the last three months

- Lipid profile, to evaluate cholesterol and triglyceride status

- CBC (complete blood count) with differential, to check for anemia or immune disorders

- High-sensitivity C-reactive protein (hsCRP), to assess degree of inflammation

- Ferritin level, to evaluate iron status

- Screening for adrenal tumors

- Food allergies

- Vitamin deficiencies, including zinc, selenium, vitamin D, and omega-3 essential fatty acids

- Heavy-metal testing

What about testing for adrenal dysfunction itself? If you are working with a conventional health-care provider, you probably won't be tested for this condition, since most conventional practitioners recognize only Addison's disease or Cushing's syndrome, two extreme adrenal disorders that are so rare their treatment is not covered in this book (though you can find out more about them in Appendix A). The tests that pick up Addison's or Cushing's won't necessarily capture other more common forms of adrenal dysfunction, though there is a test that will: *salivary cortisol testing,* which evaluates both cortisol and levels of a hormone called *DHEA.* Although conventional medical practitioners rarely use these tests, my fellow functional medical practitioners and I regularly rely on them.

However, you don't necessarily need to be formally tested for adrenal dysfunction. Once you have ruled out other potential disorders, you can simply try the suggestions in Part II and see if your symptoms resolve.

If you were to come into my office reporting one or more of the physical or psychological symptoms listed on pages 5 to 7, my ears would perk up and I'd begin to wonder if you were struggling with adrenal dysfunction. If the symptoms persisted, and especially if there was no other explanation for them, I might test your adrenal function just to be sure. And if your numbers were borderline—not quite wrong but not quite right either—I'd bring the problem to your attention, just as I'd explain that a borderline blood-sugar reading is a possible warning sign of diabetes or that a borderline blood-pressure reading could mean cardiovascular issues later on, if left unaddressed.

Conventional practitioners often take a different view. When they test you and find your readings within what's considered the "normal" range—even if at the high or low end of that range—they frequently conclude that there is no problem. Only when your numbers cross the clinically accepted threshold do they begin to treat you, and even then, they often medicate each symptom individually, with a problematic approach referred to in the literature as *polypharmacy*.

I believe there is a better way. In my view, an ounce of prevention is worth a pound of cure, and the most opportune time to start treating a problem is when the first small signs of it appear. That's the way to avoid bigger problems down the road, especially since a few little changes made in the early stages can turn the situation around. An adrenal-friendly diet, a few minutes a day spent meditating, a bit more exercise, and an altered attitude toward stress can help you to reverse every one of those trends.

The Stress Response

In recent years, the word *stress* has taken on such negative connotations, but from the body's point of view, it only means any type of demand or challenge that requires the body to expend extra energy. Getting up from your seat and walking across the room is a minor stressor, for example, because it requires more effort than remaining seated. Dinner with a sexy new romantic partner—thrilling as that may be—demands more energy than eating a bag of potato chips while sprawling on the couch. Mobilizing energy and expending it on a chosen task—rising to the occasion, in other words—is an essential part of what makes life interesting and rewarding.

But the stress response was never meant to be a permanent condition. The human body is designed to respond readily to challenges—and then to release and relax. We even have two complementary aspects of our autonomic nervous system to help us maintain that balance. (The autonomic nervous system is the aspect of our peripheral nervous system that controls the activities of our organs, glands, and various involuntary muscles, such as the cardiac and smooth muscles.)

- The *sympathetic* nervous system mobilizes energy, preparing us to meet challenges of all types. Through a number of glands and organs, including the adrenals, it causes our heart to beat faster, our blood to pump more vigorously, our blood pressure to rise, our breath to come faster and deeper, and a number of other effects designed to help us face any demanding situation.

- The *parasympathetic* nervous system stores energy, allowing the body to rest up and prepare for the next challenge. It causes our heart rate, blood pressure, and breathing to enter into a more relaxed state; and it also supports digestion and immune function so that our bodies will be in top condition next time life throws us a demand.

Our sympathetic and parasympathetic nervous systems are meant to work in tandem, like breathing in and breathing out. If you feel too wired, tired and wired, or simply exhausted, it's a good indication that you're spending too much time in challenge-meeting "sympathetic" mode, allowing too little time for "parasympathetic" recovery and restoration.

Keeping these two systems in balance used to be a matter of course. During much of human history, people relied on the sympathetic nervous system during the day, as they worked hard, defended themselves from danger, and met life's most grueling demands. They built in times for meals, rituals, prayer, and other "enforced relaxation." At night, the parasympathetic nervous system had the chance to take over. By firelight, candlelight, or lamplight, people wound down for the evening, let go of the day's work, and allowed their energy—and their adrenal reserves—to be restored.

Today, though, we live very differently from the "challenge-relax" mode for which our bodies were designed. For those of us with children, our lives look more like: *"Wake the kids and get them ready for school*—oh, my heavens, Sara, where is your other shoe? We're running late! Joshua, why didn't you tell me that you needed that permission slip signed today?—*Fight the traffic, rush to drop off the kids, hurry to work*—I know you need that right now, I'll get it for you as soon as I can—*Grab lunch while working or handling family business on the phone*—I really can't stay late tonight, I have to pick up the kids after school and the sitter just called to say she's sick . . . Well, I guess if you really need me, I can call the backup sitter—*now how am I going to pay for that? Oh, gosh, I won't have time to stop by the store*—*what is she going to feed the kids?*—" and on into the night, when we rush through dinner while attending to our children's needs, frantically do a few loads of laundry, catch up on our e-mail, make the school lunches for the next day, run the dishwasher, and maybe even finish a last-minute report or presentation.

And life without children can be similarly stressful: *"Check my e-mail before I leave for work—oh, gosh, Mom sounds pretty lonely, maybe I'd better drop by on my way home from work—Why is there so much traffic? Now I'm going to be late!*—I understand that the report needs to be redone to take the new information into account—*But why didn't they listen to me when I tried to tell them about that before I wrote it? Now my workload will be double, just because no one ever listens to me!*—Sorry, Courtney, I know we were supposed to have lunch, but I can't get away today—" The days go on and on, full of nonstop stress, frustration, and often, self-sacrifice.

For all too many of us, life is an 18-hour day of major and minor emergencies that never seem to let up. One of the keys to healing adrenal dysfunction is restoring the balance that our bodies were designed for: making sure that the exertions of our sympathetic nervous system are followed by the restoration and relaxation of our parasympathetic nervous system. Otherwise, we fall prey to the dangers of *chronic stress.*

Stress That Won't Stop

The first person to identify the effects of chronic stress was Hungarian scientist Hans Selye. From Selye's point of view, stress itself was neither good nor bad—it was simply challenging. He believed that without any stress at all, life would be pretty boring, an endless repetitive round of one familiar thing after another. Selye even dedicated his book *The Stress of Life* "to those who are not afraid to enjoy the stress of a full life . . ."

Many of my patients would be shocked by that sentence. "Enjoy stress?" they might say. "How in the world do you expect me to *enjoy* it?"

The answer lies in one word: *balance.* For stress to feel like an exhilarating challenge rather than a debilitating drain, it must always be followed by a *relaxation response.* We draw on our sympathetic nervous system to exert ourselves, and then allow our parasympathetic nervous system to help us relax—and now we're ready to face the next challenge.

But what if the stress won't let up? To answer that question, Selye created a three-stage model of the stress response, which he called the General Adaptation Syndrome, or GAS. Although we now have more biological detail than when Selye developed the GAS in the 1920s, his model is basically the one we still use.

The GAS begins with the *alarm reaction,* the jolt of energy that goes through our bodies when life places an extra demand on us. "Alarm" may be a somewhat misleading term, because this initial jolt of energy is not necessarily frightening. It's simply the extra energy we muster whenever we're faced with a challenge. A test, a speech, an unpleasant person—any of these demands require some extra effort to rise to the occasion. The challenge can also be a positive one—a date with someone we really like, the anticipation of an upcoming birthday party, the thrill of playing a game or completing an exciting project at work. Anything that requires something extra from us places an additional demand on our system, whether that "something extra" involves fun or strain—or both.

When the stress doesn't stop, however, we move into Selye's second phase, *adaptation,* in which we become accustomed to chronic stress. The body isn't really equipped for continual stress, but it does its best to rise to the occasion—day after day, month after month, year after year. Over time, the combination of insufficient sleep, never-ending demands, and the absence of genuine relaxation takes its toll.

The longer the stress continues, the greater the toll, until eventually our bodies just can't take it anymore. Our adrenal glands, charged with producing the hormones that help us rev up and rise to the occasion, lose their reserves. In Selye's final *exhaustion* phase, our adrenals are so worn out that they can't produce enough of their energizing hormones. We just don't have it in us to handle one more emergency or meet one more extra demand. This is the stage at which every little problem starts to seem like a major disaster, when your son spilling his milk or your boss giving you a disapproving look feels like the end of the world. We've all been there from time to time. But if this is your normal state *most* of the time, your system may be seriously out of balance.

Women's Stress

Although both men and women have the same basic biology when it comes to adrenal function, I sometimes think that women have an extra burden. We often put other people's needs before our own, at work as well as at home. We end up in stressful jobs where we have a lot of responsibility but very little power: waitressing, nursing, shift work, service work. When we work in offices, at any professional level, we often end up in the role of helping everyone to get along or of shouldering all the extra burdens, almost as a matter of course. We may have more than our fair share of trouble saying "no," setting limits, and taking time for ourselves. This is something I always encourage my patients to be aware of, and to make changes accordingly. (For more on how to make these changes, see Chapters 7 and 9.)

EXTRA STRESSORS

Any additional stressor puts more of a strain on your adrenal glands. Accordingly, you're at greater risk for adrenal dysfunction if you also struggle with:

- Persistent infection or chronic disease

- An eating disorder

- Smoking

- Addiction to drugs or alcohol

- Post-traumatic stress disorder

- One or more allergies, sensitivities, or types of food intolerance

- Any chronic illness, such as migraine, backache, or asthma

- Poverty, economic hardship, or simply dealing with the uncertainties of the economy

- Working a high-stress job, such as a health-care provider, emergency-room practitioner, police officer, lawyer, disaster-relief worker, midlevel manager, teacher, or shift worker

- Living or working in a noisy, demanding environment, or otherwise coping with constant noise

- Owning your own business

- Providing for your family as the sole or major breadwinner

- Dealing with sick or aging parents

- Managing work, motherhood, family responsibilities, and generally trying to "do it all"

Certainly, if we're mothers, too, we have another layer of stress. Child-rearing is one long round of large and small demands that don't really let up until your child turns 18 and leaves home—and sometimes, not even then! Starting back in those early days when our baby's cry meant that we had to go immediately and make things better, we've trained ourselves to be on constant alert, always ready to respond to the next crisis.

Caring for others is important, but so is taking care of ourselves. Our bodies were never designed to cope with constant, unremitting stress, and they will inevitably rebel if we demand that of them. Adrenal imbalance and adrenal dysfunction are cries for help—along with the painful, frustrating symptoms of weight gain, discomfort, and exhaustion.

The Health Risks of Chronic Stress

Stress isn't just unpleasant and uncomfortable—it can actually be dangerous. Numerous studies have linked chronic stress to such life-threatening conditions as cancer, heart disease, and diabetes, as well as to such problems as obesity, migraine, thyroid abnormalities, backache, and digestive disorders. Stress has also been linked to a wide variety of autoimmune disorders, either setting them off or making them worse, such as asthma, Crohn's disease, multiple sclerosis, Hashimoto's thyroiditis, antiphospholipid syndrome, and lupus. It makes sense that stress is dangerous, because none of our body's systems operate in isolation. Rather, there's a great deal of cross talk between all our systems, including adrenals, thyroid, sex hormones, gut, and brain.

I'm not trying to scare you. I am trying to support you in finding ways to ease your own version of chronic stress. Even if you are struggling with some of the life or health problems listed in the "Extra Stressors" box, you can absolutely prevent or reverse adrenal dysfunction and the other ill effects of stress, though you may have to invest some extra effort into your attempts to create downtime and genuine restoration for your body, mind, and spirit.

To help you de-stress, I offer a number of "Adrenal-Friendly Activities" throughout this book. In Chapter 9, I also share some ways to ease the historical stress that may make everything feel worse. There are also suggestions for help in the Resources section. Awareness of the problem can often feel overwhelming—but it is the first step toward empowerment and change.

Coming to Terms with Adrenal Dysfunction

We've begun to understand how chronic stress creates adrenal dysfunction, which in turn affects every one of our body's systems. For a deeper look at the interplay between stress, emotion, mind, and body, let's move on to Chapter 2.

ADRENAL-FRIENDLY ACTIVITIES:
WAYS TO BEGIN TO HEAL

- Take two minutes twice a day to meditate—or even one minute, once a day. Just inhale deeply, and then exhale while focusing on your breath.

- Massage your temples and then your earlobes—a minute each, two times a day.

- Try the following exercise in conscious breathing: Breathe in deeply, expanding your abdomen, on a count of 2. Exhale fully, also on a count of 2. Repeat, but this time use a count of 4 . . . then 6 . . . then 8 . . . then 10 . . . then 12. You can do this anywhere, but I especially like it when I'm driving, or when I'm riding on public transportation, since it's a nice, calming way to use the time.

- At the end of the day, light a lavender-scented candle and place it by your bed. Lavender helps to quiet the nerves, so take five minutes to breathe in its scent and relax.

- If you have young children, consider letting them eat first, putting them to bed, and then having an "adult meal" with your partner, a friend, or alone. Light a candle at dinner, too, turn off your cell phones, and enjoy a quiet meal.

- Consider devoting half an hour for a bath—even once a week. If you have children, make a bargain with another adult or sitter to safeguard this time.

- Buy fresh flowers and put them on your desk at work. Remember to look at them and perhaps smell them once every hour.

- Consider making time for a walk—even for 5 minutes. Try to breathe deeply and let go of work and responsibility; just let your body move.

- Keep a journal. Even if you only write a sentence or two each day, the time you take to focus on yourself could begin an important shift in focus.

- Become aware of blocks that you may have to doing these activities, and if you notice that, be gentle with yourself.

chapter two

CHRONIC STRESS AND ADRENAL DYSFUNCTION

What's Your Adrenal Stress Load?

Check all the statements that apply.

☐ When I get home, if the towels aren't perfectly folded, I have to redo them.

☐ When I entertain, I want my house to be spotless.

☐ I would like my family to help out more at home, but I can't seem to figure out how to make that happen.

☐ It's usually easier to do things myself than to ask for or accept help.

☐ If I think someone doesn't like me, I spend a lot of time worrying about it.

- [ ] Most people have it harder than I do, so I try to help other people out whenever I can.

- [ ] I find it very hard to set aside half an hour a day that is just for me.

- [ ] If everything is going well, I start to worry about what will go wrong next.

- [ ] If I have a conflict with a friend or loved one, I can't stop thinking about it.

- [ ] I'm more likely to focus on areas to be improved than on areas where I'm already strong.

- [ ] I frequently feel anxious for no apparent reason.

- [ ] If I sit in a chair with the sun behind me, no matter what time of day, I fall asleep.

My patient Katie was petite, bubbly, and in her mid-40s, with curly black hair and a raucous laugh. The owner of a local restaurant, she had helped to build the establishment into one of the town's most popular places, with a reputation for great food in the dining room and a warm, friendly atmosphere in the bar and lounge. Katie had a loving husband who adored her and a teenage stepson with whom she usually got along well.

But Katie was struggling with adrenal dysfunction, even though she had cleaned up her diet and taken all the nutrients I had suggested. Still in the early stages of adrenal fatigue, Katie's adrenal glands were working overtime, flooding her system with stress hormones. Energetic and "up" all day, Katie seemed to have endless energy, but she was creating serious hormonal imbalances that were causing her to retain weight, sleep restlessly, and struggle with an ongoing sense of anxiety. She also suffered from digestive problems, including chronic persistent diarrhea.

"I don't understand," Katie said at her next appointment. "I've done everything you've suggested, and it's true, things have improved a little. I've lost *some* weight, and I'm sleeping a *little* better. But I still have all the stomach problems, and everything is such a struggle. Things just aren't where I want them to be."

"It's terrific that you've made so many changes," I told her. "But you're putting yourself under the same pressure that you were before. Our bodies simply weren't designed for constant stress. When we ask them to keep performing and performing and don't give them time to rest, they're going to let us know that there's a problem."

Katie shook her head. "I've got a lot on my plate right now," she said. "I don't see what I can give up. Between Joe and Tyler—you know he's started living with us full-time?—and the restaurant and church, there really isn't a minute left over."

"Well, I would like you to find some way to take a few more breaks during the day," I said. "But it's not only what you do, it's how you do it. Let me ask you a question: are you constantly thinking about Joe and Tyler and the restaurant and church, even when you're 'in between' times, like driving from one place to another, or when you arrive home from work, or that last half hour before you go to bed?"

Katie looked at me in astonishment. "Of course I am! I care about my family—they're always on my mind! And my business takes everything I have to keep it going—I mean, sure, things are okay now, but three restaurants in town shut down, and I sure don't want mine to be the fourth. And at church, we're having our food drive for the soup kitchen; I can't just ignore that. . . ."

"Katie," I said to her, "I think it's wonderful that you do so much and have such a rich life—but look how upset you are right now, just thinking about all these things. Look how stressed out you are, just sitting in my office. I don't want you to give up doing anything that makes you happy or that you feel you need to do, but this is the stress that is causing the problem. No matter how many changes you make in your diet, no matter how many supplements you take, if we don't look at this stress and help you change your relationship to it, it's going to be difficult for you to solve these health problems. In fact, if nothing changes, they may very well get worse."

The Effects of a Stressful Life

Like many of my patients, Katie had a hard time accepting the relationship between the stressful life she led each day and the set of symptoms that she had come to me to heal. I think it's easier to heal ourselves and restore our bodies' balance if we can picture what's going on inside us. So let me do for you what I did for Katie and take you on a tour of your stress response.

Stress begins in the brain. As information comes in through our ears and eyes, it travels to several parts of the brain at once. One is the *cerebral cortex,* our rational, thoughtful "gray matter." Located behind the forehead, the cerebral cortex is our latest evolutionary development, enabling the complex thought, language, and memory that separates us from other animals.

Information also goes to the *amygdalas,* which are in a far older and more "primitive" part of our brains. These two small almond-shaped organs sit near each side of our head. (For practicality's sake, we usually just refer to both of them as "the amygdala.") Below them is the *brain stem,* the so-called reptile brain that handles basic animal functions, such as breathing, waking up, and falling asleep. Above the amygdala is the *limbic ring,* where our emotions are processed.

That proximity is no accident, because the amygdala gives our lives emotional weight. In his fascinating book *Emotional Intelligence,* psychologist and science journalist Daniel Goleman describes a man who had his amygdala surgically removed to control severe seizures. As a result, the man "became completely uninterested in people, preferring to sit in isolation with no human contact." He could recognize his loved ones. He just didn't care about them.

Think about what this means. When we get information from the outside world, it goes to two different processing centers. One, the cerebral cortex, is logical and language-based. It tries to make a rational assessment about how great a danger or how daunting a challenge we might be facing. Based on that assessment, it gives instructions to the body to mobilize energy as necessary: "That car looks like it isn't going to slow down—change lanes!" "Jessica will be upset if I don't pick up her favorite cereal from the store on the way home." "It will be easier to get out in the morning if I make the lunches now— I'd better find that permission slip tonight or Leo won't have it tomorrow—" That's the cerebral cortex talking, instructing us on how to meet the major emergencies and minor challenges of our lives.

Meanwhile, the same information goes to the emotional, impulsive amygdala. It will also decide—with all the intense emotion of which we are capable—whether or not we're in danger or are facing a major challenge. It also has the power to instruct the body to mobilize energy: "Car—*danger!*" "Jessica—tantrum—aargh! *Stop her!*" "Busy, busy—*hurry!*"

As you can see, both the cerebral cortex and the amygdala make decisions about when we need to mobilize energy. They implement those decisions through the sympathetic nervous system, which, as we saw in Chapter 1, revs us up. Both the rational cerebral cortex and the impulsive amygdala send signals to the *hypothalamus,* a key portion of our brain that sits at the base of our skull, even deeper within our "primitive" brain stem than the amygdala.

The hypothalamus has many functions, but for the moment let's focus on its role in mobilizing energy. When either the cerebral cortex or the amygdala identifies a potential threat, a major task, or any demand that requires effort, it notifies the hypothalamus.

Through a complicated chemical reaction that I'll describe in a moment, the hypothalamus instructs the sympathetic nervous system to mobilize our energy for action.

Significantly, this process works pretty much the same way for any type of stress—positive or negative. Our bodies will respond similarly whether we have just identified an angry client, a fascinating topic for a report, or a thrilling new romantic prospect. Whether we are angry, happy, scared, or simply confused, our brain says, "We need energy," and our body responds.

Ideally, our cerebral cortex and our amygdala know how to distinguish between minor and major challenges. If we're about to return a phone call from that sexy new love interest, we might need only a little extra energy; when we actually go on our first date, we may be far more excited. If we have to open a tightly wrapped DVD, we need only a little extra energy; if we need to clean out the garage, which hasn't been touched in years, we may need to muster a great deal more.

Sometimes, though, we expend far more energy than we really need to, perhaps because our emotions take over. Even though we know it's "not such a big deal," we can't sleep for three nights running before giving a major speech at work. Our daughter accidentally tips her bowl of applesauce onto our just-washed kitchen floor, and we feel as though the bottom has dropped out of our world. Last night's date calls back the next morning, and just at the sight of the caller ID, our heart starts racing and we lose our appetite. Whether or not we've correctly calibrated our response, some part of our brain has conveyed to our hypothalamus that we need energy, and suddenly our sympathetic nervous system is flooding our body with stress hormones. Sweaty palms, pounding heart, and rising blood pressure are the result.

How exactly does the message get out? After being alerted by our rational and/or emotional brain, the hypothalamus releases CRH, short for *corticotropin-releasing hormone*. (Don't worry, you're never going to have to remember that name.) Our CRH travels to another gland, the *pituitary,* where it activates another hormone you won't have to remember: ACTH, or *adrenocorticotropic hormone*. ACTH, in turn, stimulates your *adrenal glands*. This pathway—hypothalamus to pituitary to adrenals—is known as the *hypothalamic-pituitary-adrenal axis,* or HPA axis for short.

Two key stress hormones are *adrenaline* (also known as epinephrine) and *noradrenaline* (a.k.a. norepinephrine). Each has complicated roles to play in the stress response, but adrenaline, at least, has given its name to the famous "adrenaline rush"—the excitement of confronting a life-or-death challenge and coming out victorious. Soldiers in combat, nurses in the emergency room, and vacationers on a roller coaster all experience something of this thrill, an exhilarating fear in which high stakes are part of the "high."

Another key stress hormone is *cortisol*—and that is a name I *would* like you to remember. One of cortisol's key jobs is to sustain our blood-sugar levels when we have to "fight or flee." After all, for our early human ancestors, most challenges probably came in the form of a physical demand, and so our muscles needed all the blood-sugar-based energy they could get, as did our brain, heart, and lungs. Cortisol to the rescue!

If stress is short-term and followed by relaxation, there's no problem: cortisol might drive our blood-sugar levels up, but then other chemicals, released by the soothing parasympathetic nervous system, will drive them down again. When we're stressed all the time, though, with few real breaks, cortisol keeps our blood-sugar levels permanently high. This plays havoc with our metabolism and can make it nearly impossible to lose weight—or to keep from gaining. (For more on stress, cortisol, and weight, see below.)

The stress response doesn't stop there. Cortisol and another stress hormone, *aldosterone,* help our kidneys reabsorb sodium. That process helps to conserve electrolytes and water in our bloodstream, so that—when we are fighting or fleeing—extra blood can be more easily pumped into critical organs and tissues. In other words, our blood pressure goes up and, if the stress is chronic, we may have problems with fluid retention.

Besides taking orders from the cerebral cortex and the amygdala, the hypothalamus also responds to immune signals and to pain. So if we're struggling with an autoimmune condition, such as asthma, rheumatoid arthritis, or chronic allergies (which may themselves be triggered and/or intensified by either stress or HPA imbalance), our stress levels rise accordingly. Our stress levels will also rise in response to chronic pain, environmental sensitivities, or any other combination of physical and psychological stressors, such as an eating disorder. Indeed, any emotional or physical challenge can "alarm" our hypothalamus, setting off a stress response that can eventually become chronic.

As you can see, much of the stress response is intended to gear up our bodies to respond to immediate physical challenges. In modern times, though, we might not need our muscles to respond to life's demands. Instead, we might be wrestling with a knotty problem ("The deadline just got moved up!" "I can't pay all my bills!"), agonizing over a relationship issue ("He just canceled our date!" "I called his hotel room and some woman answered—is he having an affair?"), or coping with our children ("Brian just got an F in English!" "Cynthia is the only girl in her class who didn't get invited to that party!").

So now our body faces two potential problems. First, our stress response has revved us up for physical activity that we're probably not going to undertake. Fleeing a tiger or fighting an enemy would require high blood-sugar levels and higher blood pressure, because our muscles and tissues need extra support. Coping with a distressed child or a frustrating partner doesn't require the same physical exertion, yet we've prepared our bodies to respond anyway, with no physical release in sight. (Please don't read this and run right out to the gym! Lack of physical release may be part of how the problem started, but intense exercise may *not* be the right way to address your *current* state. I'll help you figure out the levels of exercise that are correct for you *now* in Chapter 7.)

Second, our ancestors knew when the challenge was over—when the enemy had been defeated or the predator evaded. But as Katie found, *our* level of stress may never go down. Instead of the healthy challenge-relax model that we identified in Chapter 1, in which the sympathetic nervous system is well balanced by the parasympathetic nervous system, many of us today are living in constant "high-alert" mode, with no real chance to let go. Instead of the *acute* stress for which our stress response is designed, our body is living under *chronic* stress—something it was never intended to do.

As you can see, our approach to stress intensifies the immediate pressures that we often face, turning acute stress into chronic stress. In his brilliant book, *Why Zebras Don't Get Ulcers,* Stanford neuroscientist Robert Sapolsky explains that zebras worry only about what's right in front of them. When a lion chases them, they fear it—and run away. But when no lion is in sight, they don't continually worry, *What if the lion comes back?* Nor do they say to themselves, *What if I'm not strong enough or smart enough or worthy enough to escape the lion?* Or, *None of the other zebras will like me if I'm not good at running away from the lion. I'll be all alone.* Or, *Remember last week how the lion almost got me? What was* wrong *with me? Why can't I ever run faster?* As a result, zebras don't experience chronic stress. They stress only about what happens to them in the present.

Most humans handle stress very differently. We live in a state of chronic stress in which real-life challenges are magnified by fears, anxieties, worries, and memories, creating a constant state of inescapable tension. We try to please the other people in our lives, or to live up to our own high standards, or to reach some kind of ideal state in which all the deadlines are met and all the children are happy and all the work has been done. And behind those real-life challenges may be the echoes of our parents, who perhaps were angry or frustrated or sad or resentful or short-tempered or addicted or otherwise struggling with challenges of their own, and who, without intending to, left us feeling as though nothing we do will ever be good enough and no life we build will ever be quite as safe and secure as we would like it to be.

In other words, stress has two aspects: *real-life* and *historical*. It's *historical* stress that tends to remain constantly at the back of our minds, even when real-life challenges have ended.

The Problem of Perception

When I suggested to Katie that her own perceptions and emotional history might be part of the puzzle, her first response was to disagree.

"Look, I love Tyler, but he's not the easiest kid to take care of, especially now. He loves Joe and me, but he misses his mom, and sometimes he takes it out on us. That's not me—it's him! He just yells at me for no reason, like 'You're not my mom! You can't tell me what to do!' The restaurant is hard. That's the economy—it isn't me. And don't get me started about those women at church!"

I agreed with everything Katie said, but I still thought she had some options she wasn't considering. Her circumstances were what they were, but her *perception* of those circumstances could potentially change. If her perception changed, her stress levels might change as well.

Let me give you an example of how our perceptions affect our stress levels. Suppose you're driving to work and you're running a bit late. You're already on edge because your boss has reprimanded you twice this week for not being on time, plus you have a ton of work waiting for you.

Suddenly, out of nowhere, a speeding car cuts you off, dashes through traffic, barely avoids several collisions, and runs a red light. You're terrified, shaken—and very, very angry. "Selfish creep—how dare he put the rest of us in danger like that? Now I've missed the light *and* I'll be late! That rotten guy, who does he think he is?" Your anger rises, your stress levels go up, and you feel more frustrated than ever. *Everybody gets their way but me,* you think. *They just break the rules any time they want to, while I have to sit here like a good girl doing the right thing—and now* I'm *going to get in trouble! And when I think about how much I have to do this morning . . .*

Now suppose someone told you that the speeding car was driven by a father whose child had lost consciousness. There wasn't time to call an ambulance, so he's rushing his son to the hospital, desperate to save his life. Your anger, frustration, and resentment instantly melt away, to be replaced with compassion and concern. *That poor guy . . . I hope his kid's all right. . . . He must be frantic. . . . I hope it all works out okay. . . . Thank God my own kids are all right. Boy, I'm going to give them all an extra hug when I see them tonight. . . .*

The events of the morning—the speeding car, the potential lateness to your job, the mountain of work that's waiting for you—are all exactly the same. What has changed is your *perception* of events. Instead of viewing the speeding car as an unfair intrusion, you view it as a sad necessity. Instead of responding with anger and frustration, you respond with compassion and perhaps gratitude for your own good fortune. You may feel shaken and a bit sad, but you don't feel stressed. Just one little shift in perception has completely altered your response.

I'm not suggesting that you become a mindless optimist or that you simply ignore problems that are all too pressing and real. But I do believe there is a powerful connection between how we look at our lives and how stressed we tend to feel.

In Katie's case, one of the biggest challenges came in her responses to Tyler, her 13-year-old stepson. Now let me be the first to say it: raising teenagers *can* be stressful. However, there are ways that our perceptions might make things easier or harder. Whenever Tyler cried out to Katie, "You're not my *real* mom!" Katie felt her heart sink. Her entire body seized up in a fight-or-flight response that lasted far longer than the initial argument. Long after Tyler had stormed up to his room and started playing video games, Katie continued to stew. How dare he talk to her that way? Didn't he know she was doing the best she could? Why didn't he appreciate all she was doing for him?

Underneath the anger was a deep feeling of fear: No, she wasn't Tyler's real mom— maybe that meant she really *couldn't* take care of him. What if she couldn't help him the way he needed? What would Joe think of her? Would Joe leave her? What was wrong with her, anyway?

In fact, Katie's responses—especially the feelings of fear and inadequacy—were not really about Tyler and Joe. They had far more to do with her parents and her own childhood. "What's wrong with you—why can't you do anything right?" was something Katie's own mother had shouted to her many, many times. When Tyler shouted something similar, Katie wasn't just feeling the stress of being 40-something with a frustrated teenage stepson. She was feeling the guilt, shame, and panic of a little girl with an angry mom.

Moreover, Katie's own father had left the family when Katie turned 13, so her fears that Joe would also leave her were fed by her early experience with her father. Whenever I asked Katie whether Joe might really leave her, she always said, "Oh, don't be silly, I know he's in it for the long haul! He always says he couldn't live without me, and I know he means it."

But Katie's sensible words did little to calm her fears. Her rational mind in the cerebral cortex understood that Joe would stay. But her amygdala in the emotion-processing limbic ring *knew* he was going to leave. Her amygdala communicated with her hypothalamus, which communicated along the HPA axis with her adrenals—and constant floods of cortisol were the result.

This is how real-life stress is magnified by historical stress. Katie's actual fight with Tyler had lasted maybe five minutes. But the fears, worries, guilt, anger, and feelings of inadequacy went on for hours. And all that time, Katie's amygdala was signaling her HPA axis, cuing her adrenals to send out cortisol and other stress hormones. Her blood pressure was up and her blood sugar was rising, preparing for a physical exertion that never actually came.

Katie didn't need those stress hormones to rise to an emotional challenge, let alone a physical one—Tyler had long since stopped playing video games and gone to bed. But Katie was wide awake and full of stress, her limbic system signaling *threat, threat, threat* as she wrestled with her feelings. Her hypothalamus heard the threat message loud and clear, so it sent messages along the HPA axis instructing her adrenals to keep flooding her system. As we'll see a little later on, the resulting excess of cortisol had serious effects on Katie's weight, digestion, mood, and overall health.

In Chapter 9, I'll share some suggestions for how you might rework some of your perceptions and heal these historical wounds—suggestions that might greatly help you to reduce your stress. For now, let's just remember that the way we view the world often creates a state of chronic stress. And since chronic stress is at the root of adrenal dysfunction, if we're going to rebalance our adrenals, we must address our stress.

Our Impulsive Amygdala

"Act first and ask questions later."

That frantic phrase might be the amygdala's motto, because fast, impulsive action is its specialty. Although our rational cerebral cortex looks for a complete and sensible version of events, our amygdala is designed to get just a brief impression—*fast.*

Suppose you were walking in the woods with your daughter, and a snake seemed to cross your path. The information would be sent to your amygdala, which would instantly signal "Danger!" to your HPA axis. With all the strength and energy that your body has developed to meet emergencies, you'd leap out of the way and pull your child with you—all before you're consciously aware of what you've done.

Maybe when your thinking brain kicks in, you'd realize that the "snake" was only a branch, or that it was a harmless snake rather than a poisonous one. But if it *had* been a poisonous snake, your thinking brain might have been too late. The amygdala helps you take quick, impulsive action, literally before you realize what you're doing.

How does our impulsive, reactive side manage to take over so quickly, while our thoughtful, rational brain always seems to show up a little late? That's because information arrives at our amygdala twice as quickly as it reaches the cerebral cortex. Literally before we have a chance to think things through, our amygdala has already received the sensory data and come to its own conclusions.

Then, a few beats later, our cerebral cortex gets the information and weighs in. Whereas initially, our amygdala simply shouts, *"Snake!"* our cerebral cortex explains, "That's not a snake, it's a branch!" If our boss comes into the office and says, "I don't know why things can't get done more quickly around here," our amygdala screams, "He's out to get me!" Then, a bit later, our cerebral cortex might say, "Actually, he wasn't even talking to me, he was talking to Mary." When our daughter cries, our amygdala wails right along: "She hates me!" But hopefully our cerebral cortex has the chance to comment, "She doesn't *really* hate me; she's just a hungry five-year-old who missed her nap." In other words, our amygdala is constantly ready to shout, "Danger! Danger! Danger!" before our cerebral cortex has the chance to express a different perspective: "No danger here, just calm down—everything is actually fine!"

As you can see, one of the amygdala's most important jobs is to protect us and our loved ones when we don't have time to think things through. It actually has direct access to our hypothalamus, which, as we saw in the snake example, enables it to set in motion our fight-or-flight response at top speed via the HPA axis.

But that hair-trigger emergency-response system can be a double-edged sword. Our amygdala does a great job when the perceived threat is simple, clear, and in the present. But it's not nearly as useful when the danger we perceive is an emotional one, a situation that may require thought, analysis, and a careful sorting-through of all our different options. If Katie needed to save Tyler from a snake, her amygdala would help her snatch him out of harm's way. But if Katie is fighting with Tyler over an emotional issue, her impulsive, anxious, intense response may not be the best way to handle things.

Our amygdala can be especially problematic when present-day stressors remind us of events from the past: the boss's voice that sounds like Daddy's, the friend's reproach that reminds us of Mom. Suddenly, thanks to our amygdala, those similarities can trigger a kind of emotional flashback that puts us right back into childhood, with all the panic, fear, and sorrow that we felt the first time we were yelled at, or the first time we made Mommy cry. That intense wave of emotion feels out of our control—and in many ways, it is. When we feel panicked or miserable or enraged even though we know we "shouldn't," we are actually reliving our emotional memories, through the amygdala. Different types of memory are stored in different parts of the brain, but our *emotional* memory lives in the amygdala. So when an event reminds us of something from our past, the amygdala releases the memory in all its vivid intensity.

We've all had this experience at one time or another. A smell makes us unaccountably happy—then we realize that it's the smell of salt, and it reminds us of that wonderful time Mommy took us to the beach. A song makes us suddenly miserable—and then we remember that it was playing when our teenage boyfriend broke up with us. Sensory data is linked to many different types of memories, and they can carry a strong emotional resonance that can flood us with surprising vividness.

Oftentimes that emotional memory operates independently of our rational brain. If the event happened when we were too young to consciously remember it, our bodies may still hold the sorrow or the joy. If an event at any age was too traumatic, we may deny its importance or even "forget" it to protect ourselves—but our bodies and emotions continue to remember. We carry many strong emotions without necessarily knowing what caused them—and therefore without being able to consciously control them.

Just because we can't understand our emotions doesn't mean that they don't have power over us. Quite the contrary. Our emotional memories can be extremely powerful, especially when something happens to trigger our amygdala into another state of panic.

For example, Katie had grown up with a boisterous alcoholic father who frequently came home drunk and engaged in loud shouting matches with her mother. If he got angry enough, he'd strike out physically, never actually beating Katie but sometimes giving her a slap or a shove. For Katie, therefore, a loud voice signified *danger,* and her amygdala learned to kick into high gear as soon as the decibel count crossed a certain threshold. Whenever a man raised his voice around her, stress hormones flooded her body, particularly cortisol.

Katie's husband, Joe, was also a loud, boisterous man, but he wouldn't hurt a fly and he'd certainly never hurt Katie. Still, when Joe got annoyed, he did raise his voice—and Katie's entire body went into panic mode. With the same instant impulsive response she would have used to jump out of the way of a dangerous snake (or something that *looked* like a dangerous snake), she jumped to do anything, at all costs, to keep the peace.

Katie's cerebral cortex knew perfectly well that Joe would never shove or slap her. But her amygdala didn't know that. It signaled her HPA axis to respond to Joe's loudness just as it had responded to her father's shouting: with a racing heart, rising blood pressure, interrupted digestion, and all the other elements of the stress response meant to help us fight or flee. Katie's default fight-or-flight mode, learned from years of growing up with her father, was to put an enormous amount of panicked energy into trying to calm Joe down, even as she lived in constant fear of his anger. All those stressful emotions kept Katie's adrenal glands working overtime—and adrenal dysfunction was the result.

As Katie discovered, simply understanding the problem intellectually wasn't enough. That's because understanding happened in the more advanced portion of her brain—her thoughtful cerebral cortex. Panic, though, began in her emotional, impulsive amygdala. For Katie to stop stressing her adrenals—and for her adrenals to stop flooding her body with cortisol—she needed to engage in the kind of emotional reprogramming that could reach the primitive part of her brain. (I'll explain how to do that reprogramming in Chapter 9.)

POSSIBLE EFFECTS OF ADRENAL DYSFUNCTION

Anxiety	Hypoglycemia/blood-sugar fluctuations
Autoimmune disorders	Immune dysregulation
Chronic fatigue syndrome	Infertility
Decreased sex drive	Insomnia
Depression	Mood swings
Fatigue	Palpitations
Feeling faint	PMS
Fibromyalgia	Recurring infections
Fluid retention	Thyroid abnormalities
Foggy brain	Type 2 diabetes
Frequent muscle aches and pains	Weight gain
GI dysfunction	Weight retention

The Dangers of Chronic Stress

Katie was beginning to understand how the combination of *real-life stress* and *historical stress* was creating *chronic stress*. But I also wanted her to see how the constantly high levels of stress hormones were affecting her entire body.

When the hypothalamus sends its "alarm" message along the HPA axis, several stress hormones are ultimately released. We've already looked at the way cortisol floods the system, keeping our blood sugar high. Along with cortisol, the adrenals release *epinephrine* (also known as *adrenaline*) and *norepinephrine* (also known as *noradrenaline*). As a result your heart beats faster, your blood pumps harder, and your breath comes faster and deeper. In other words, your heart begins to stress and your blood pressure goes up.

Again, this would be a useful reaction if you were actually facing a vigorous physical challenge requiring fight or flight. And it would not necessarily be a damaging reaction if, after the crisis had passed, your body could return to a more relaxed state.

When stress is chronic, however, there is no relaxed state. The hormones signaling your heart to beat faster and your blood pressure to rise remain in your system—and your heart and blood vessels do their best to respond.

At the same time, your stomach and gastrointestinal systems are getting messages of their own. After all, if you're going to fight or flee, you don't have time to stop and eat a sandwich. And digestion is far less important than getting blood and energy to those all-important muscles. As a result, your stomach under stress has a harder time contracting, and a harder time emptying, leading you to feel full and bloated. Your colon, by contrast, hurries to empty itself—no use carrying all that extra waste during a fight or flight. That means you don't absorb nutrients or water very well. Meanwhile, the extra activity of your colon can cause your bowel to become inflamed. You might also get diarrhea.

Again, these would be fine as temporary reactions. If the stress persists, however, your body starts to rebel. The balance between the stimulating sympathetic nervous system and the calming parasympathetic nervous system is disturbed, and this keeps your stomach from contracting and emptying itself as it should. This is exactly what happened to Katie. As I explained to her, she was potentially setting herself up for bowel dysfunction. People with Crohn's disease—another type of problem with the colon—find their symptoms become much worse in response to chronic stress.

A high-adrenaline lifestyle can also create instability in a woman's moods and emotions. Scientific research has linked anxiety and depression with the high levels of cortisol that result from a life lived on the edge. Over time, as the adrenals become progressively less able to sustain high levels of adrenaline, both the buzz and the anxiety generated by this hormone wear off and the woman is left feeling flat, with the predominant symptom of depression. So by living with chronic stress, Katie was potentially setting herself up for depression, as well as digestive problems.

Our digestive problems also become problems for our mood and emotions. That's because one of the key hormones produced in our gut is serotonin, the "antidepressant" hormone that is crucial to our sense of optimism, self-esteem, self-confidence, and well-being. Many antidepressants are SSRIs, a type of medication that combats depression by preventing the reuptake of serotonin, thus keeping more serotonin circulating in the system. But if you suffer from digestive problems, as Katie did, your ability to manufacture serotonin may be compromised, since two-thirds of serotonin is produced in the gut. So by living with chronic stress, Katie was potentially setting herself up for depression.

An imbalance between the sympathetic and the parasympathetic nervous systems can also affect the body parts that regulate and support our immune system: the thymus, spleen, lymph nodes, bone marrow, and an immune system feature embedded in the gut known as intestinal Peyer's patches. Through a complicated series of biochemical reactions, the chronic flooding of the body with stress hormones acts to suppress the immune response, making us more vulnerable to disease, infection, and cancer.

Cortisol compromises our immune system in another way. As I explained in my earlier book, *The Core Balance Diet, telomeres* are the tiny clocks that cap the DNA within each cell and regulate that cell's biological age. Whenever a cell divides, its telomeres get shorter, which in effect ages both it and you. An enzyme called *telomerase* has a special protective function for the telomeres in your cells, including your immune cells. Cortisol, however, suppresses your immune cells' ability to manufacture telomerase. As a result, the body's defenses are suppressed, and the immune system is weakened.

Unfortunately, that's not all. When the HPA axis is disturbed, a number of other hormones are thrown out of balance. Thyroid—influencing energy, mood, metabolism, and body temperature—can be affected. So can growth hormone, which also affects energy, mood, and metabolism. Our sex hormones are thrown out of balance as well, especially as we progress through perimenopause and into menopause. Although sex hormones are manufactured in the ovaries, some small amounts are made by the adrenal glands as well. During perimenopause and menopause, the adrenals start to play a more important role, producing some estrogen, progesterone, testosterone, DHEA, pregnenolone, and androstenedione. As we age, the ovaries begin to shut down, decreasing their production of these hormones. When healthy, the adrenals can fill in the gaps by orchestrating the production of these sex hormones—but if they're shunting their energy into stress-hormone production, they don't have adequate reserves to fulfill this task. Difficulties with perimenopause and menopause are the result.

Meanwhile, throughout our lives, our testosterone is manufactured in the adrenals as well as in the ovaries. Although testosterone is considered the "male hormone," we women have it, too, and it's responsible for a great deal of our libido and our drive in general. So we need our adrenals to help keep us well supplied with "male" and "female" sex hormones, or we risk such symptoms as lowered sex drive and a general feeling of listlessness. Disturbing the HPA axis has profound consequences indeed.

Another aspect of the HPA axis involves aldosterone, a hormone that helps to regulate our sodium-potassium balance and our retention or release of fluids. Like cortisol, aldosterone is supposed to peak at around 8 A.M. and reach a low between midnight and

4 A.M. But when we're stressed, ACTH, the same hormone that stimulates the release of cortisol, leads to the release of aldosterone as well.

If high levels of cortisol remain in the system for 24 hours or so, the cells that produce aldosterone lose their sensitivity to ACTH. As a result, chronic stress often leads to the *under*production of aldosterone—the symptoms of which include low blood pressure, bloating and water retention, electrolyte imbalance, increased thirst, general muscle weakness and lethargy, and sometimes a craving for salt.

Another key group of adrenal hormones are called the *glucocorticoids,* which help metabolize proteins, carbohydrates, and, to a lesser extent, fats. In the right quantities, glucocorticoids help us fight allergies and *inflammation*, the response of our tissues to infection or injury. So the anti-inflammatory properties of glucocorticoids are extremely beneficial to our health. In fact, a form of this biochemical, known as *prednisone,* is often used to treat rheumatoid arthritis.

While acute inflammation is often necessary to help the body heal, *chronic low-grade systemic inflammation* can create myriad problems of its own, including autoimmune conditions, diabetes, heart disease, and cancer, among others. When glucocorticoid levels remain too high for too long—as they tend to do under stress—then they actually *fuel* inflammation. Now we're at risk for the very conditions that glucocorticoids could once help protect us from.

Chronic stress also affects our mood and our behavior. Animals who have been injected with CRH—the hormone that the hypothalamus uses to set off the stress response—have been seen to:

- Move in an agitated fashion

- Startle more easily

- Fight more often

- Lose interest in eating

- Begin avoiding unfamiliar and threatening places

- Show symptoms of clinical depression: lack of interest in pleasurable activities; changes in appetite, weight, and sleep; fatigue; and self-destructive behavior.

In other words, as I explained to Katie, chronic stress ultimately affects just about every one of our body's systems, with particularly intense effects on our thyroid, digestive system, and sex hormones. Although we're used to speaking of the HPA axis, I've come to follow the broader view of functional-medicine pioneer Dr. Jeffrey Bland in considering the entire HPATGG axis: hypothalamic-pituitary-adrenal-thyroid-gut-gonad, because our bodies are not really compartmentalized—ultimately, the body is all one big system. That system is set up to handle temporary acute stress—but not continual chronic stress. Adrenal dysfunction is one result of chronic stress, but sadly, it is not the only one.

Growing Up Stressed

It's bad enough when adults live with chronic stress that overstimulates their HPA axis. But when infants and children have to endure unremitting stress, the effects are even more severe: they begin to underproduce growth hormone and other key biochemicals in a variant of the condition sometimes referred to as "failure to thrive." Such children may not gain weight even when they consume ample calories, because their systems don't have the hormones they need to grow.

The ill effects of childhood stress continue on into adulthood. Studies have shown that the early loss of a parent, physical abuse, and sexual abuse during childhood all create an increased risk of major depression during adulthood. And a history of major depression contributes in turn to a loss of bone density, cardiovascular risk (including increased risk of stroke, blood clots, heart attack, and congestive heart failure), and a host of other disorders.

When the HPA axis is overstimulated in childhood, it often continues to remain out of balance into adulthood. As a result, childhood abuse creates a greater risk of adult anxiety disorders, panic disorder, post-traumatic stress disorder, and possibly also suicide. Women who were abused as children are also more likely to become obese as a result of the excessive stress hormones that flood their bodies. I'll say more on the connection between stress and obesity in the next section. Abused women also have a greater tendency toward PMS, asthma, spastic colitis, and dysmenorrhea (painful menstrual periods). People who have experienced childhood trauma are also at risk for immune disorders, including increased vulnerability to the common cold. And they may be at risk for increased blood pressure and other cardiovascular problems.

If you've experienced high levels of childhood stress, what does this mean for you? First, congratulate yourself on having gotten to the place where you're now seeking greater understanding and new solutions. Second, understand that your health problems—especially with regard to adrenal dysfunction—have their roots in your early experiences as well as your current ones. Third, look at Chapter 9 and at the Resources section for support in moving forward and healing these childhood wounds. It can be done—and by reading this, you've taken an important step.

Chronic Stress and Weight Gain

One of the most frustrating effects of excess cortisol for many of my patients is the way it contributes to weight retention and/or weight gain. Woman after woman has sat in my office, describing her increasingly Spartan diet and her even more demanding exercise plan, only to find that she either didn't lose weight or actually gained it.

As I explained in *The Core Balance Diet,* one of the ways your body compensates for unremitting stress is to go into survival mode by switching metabolic gears. This harkens back to the days of our feast-or-famine past, when "stress" truly meant life-threatening danger, and unremitting stress might well have meant lack of access to food and increased need for physical exertion.

I like to picture our ancestors migrating across the African desert, or perhaps trekking through uncharted forests in cold northern lands. Day after day, their energy was mobilized for extra effort, as they trudged through the snowy woods or across the hot sands. The women had to make sure that the children could keep up, and besides the physical stress of migration they also must have felt a great deal of fear—for their children, their families, and themselves. Most likely there wasn't enough to eat, and so their bodies responded to this constant stress by holding on to every bit of fat they could.

When I explained this to Katie, she was at first relieved to understand what had happened to her, then frustrated by what she had just learned. "So how am I supposed to tell my body to switch gears and lose weight?" she asked me. "I know the extra weight is causing health problems of its own, and it's sure making me *feel* lousy."

Katie was certainly right about the health problems. In addition to the increased risk of heart disease and diabetes, the excess fat itself posed a problem. We've recently come to learn that body fat is not an inert substance but is instead metabolically active. All those extra fat cells contribute to the production of certain kinds of cytokines, biochemicals that promote inflammation, which, as we just saw, can contribute to a number of disorders.

The solution, as I explained to Katie, was not to further stress the body by reducing calories or increasing exercise. Instead, an adrenal-friendly diet, herbal supplements, and the right kind of exercise were called for, along with efforts to heal the root cause of the problem: the chronic stress that was signaling her body to remain in a constant state of emergency.

I suggested to Katie some of the adrenal-friendly activities I listed in Chapter 1, along with some of the other solutions to be found in the "Adrenal-Friendly Activities" boxes offered throughout this book. Like most of my patients, she was delighted to find that even small changes could make a big difference in the way she felt.

Learning to Release

Once Katie accepted that chronic stress was at the root of her problem, she applied her characteristic energy and drive to addressing it, using the techniques I've laid out throughout this book. Over time, Katie learned to release much of her chronic stress while still maintaining her ambition and determination. Her success stands as a testament to the power we can unleash when we commit to changing our relationship to stress.

ADRENAL-FRIENDLY ACTIVITIES: WAYS TO BEGIN TO HEAL

- *Put your hand on your heart.* Neural cells around our heart become activated during stress. This simple exercise can send them a calming message. Try it once or twice a day, for one or two minutes at a time.

  1. Place your hand over your heart.

  2. Inhale and exhale slowly.

  3. Think about a person who loves you, a favorite place, or a happy memory while you continue to take deep, slow breaths.

- *Smile consciously.* Psychologist Paul Ekman has discovered that facial expressions can actually produce corresponding feelings; in other words, we feel what our faces communicate. Because of the way we are wired, smiling can evoke positive feelings in us by stimulating our autonomic nervous system to release endorphins, opiates (natural painkillers), and serotonin, the "anti-depressant" hormone that sustains our sense of well-being, optimism, and self-esteem. If you hate the idea of forcing yourself to smile, hold a pencil between your teeth for one or two minutes twice a day. That will also activate your smile muscles, leading your heart rate to decrease and causing you to feel happier and calmer.

- *Tap your thymus.* The thymus is a key part of your immune system, as it produces the T-cells that fight off infections. Tapping the center of your chest, where your thymus is located, stimulates the thymus to produce more T-cells by drawing blood and energy into the thymus. Tapping also helps massage the lungs, heart, bronchial tubes, and throat. Make your hand into a fist and strike yourself firmly but gently in the center of your chest, right between your breasts. Pause, then strike twice more, more lightly. Repeat the sequence—strong tap, pause, two light taps—for up to five minutes. Since your thymus is most active about 90 minutes after you fall asleep, ideally, you would tap first thing in the morning or about half an hour before bedtime, but you can use this exercise at any time during the day as a way to combat stress.

- *Practice awareness.* Simply start to become aware of the things that cause you to feel stressed. Now that you've read the first part of this book, you may start to hear some echoes from your childhood. Or you may suddenly notice resources in your life that you haven't been taking advantage of—opportunities for finding time for yourself or for enlisting help and support at home or at work. So often we expect too much from ourselves, and the effort to de-stress ironically adds even more stress to our already overburdened lives. If that's how you feel, please, give yourself a break. Start from where you are, don't judge yourself, and don't ask yourself to do anything more than become aware.

- *Salute yourself.* Believe me, I know all too well how hard it can be to focus on the positive when all you see is how much you *haven't* done. But let me encourage you to "flip the script" and give yourself huge pats on the back that you've even picked up this book, that you are even willing to entertain the possibility that some things in your life need to change. Kudos to you for taking the first step of simply reading these words! Now that you've taken that first step, who knows what others might follow?

WHAT'S YOUR
ADRENAL PROFILE?

Jasmine is a high-powered executive in the finance industry whose days start with early-morning breakfast meetings and end in late-night drinks with clients. In her late 30s, she's proud of how much she's accomplished, and she genuinely loves her job. She's always full of energy and makes sure that an hour at the gym is part of her daily sched-ule, but she's recently started gaining weight. She's also become increasingly irritable, and she's begun to notice some disturbing symptoms: raging PMS, painful periods, low-ered sex drive, and thinning hair. Jasmine has always struggled with allergies, and as a child she suffered from asthma. Lately it seems that her allergies are acting up worse than ever, especially first thing in the morning and at the end of a long day. She's also noticed that the bleach she uses to whiten her sheets has started making her eyes water.

When Tracy's alarm goes off in the morning, she can barely drag herself out of bed to make breakfast for her two kids. A social worker in her early 30s, she's come to dread the mornings: no matter how many cups of coffee she mainlines, she can't seem to wake up. The afternoons are slightly better, but Tracy really dreads her "four o'clock low" as well. She perks up at dinnertime, just as her husband and children are winding down for the night. And by 10 P.M., when her husband is sound asleep, Tracy is totally wired. The only one awake in the house, she finds herself anxiously counting her worries: bills, her daughter's poor grades, a troublesome client at work. To calm herself, she fixes a sweet nighttime snack and watches TV, often until 1 A.M. or 2 A.M. Then, the next morning, the cycle starts all over again. Sometimes Tracy thinks the only relief she gets is when she's sick—but she hates being sick. This winter, she's had three colds, an episode of stomach flu, and a long-lasting bout of bronchitis. She also suffers from chronic lower-back pain, although, she tells me, she's "used to that."

Rosario is a single mother in her mid-40s who works as a customer-service representative for the local cable company. She's about 30 pounds over her ideal weight and keeps promising herself to exercise, but she never seems to find the time—or the energy. A botched knee operation five or six years ago has left her with severe knee pain, which comes and goes during the day but which never really leaves. Every morning she wakes up at 5:30, makes breakfast for her eight-year-old son, heads off to work, brings her son home, makes dinner, helps him with his homework, and falls into bed at 9:30, exhausted. On weekends she parks her son in front of the TV or arranges a playdate for him and sleeps as much as she can. Rosario used to date, go out to clubs with her girlfriends, and sing in a local choir. One by one, she's given up everything but the bare minimum, because she's so exhausted. No matter how much sleep she gets, she feels as though she can barely drag herself through the day.

Stress and the Allostatic Load

One of the challenges of understanding adrenal dysfunction is that the same condition can take so many different forms. Rosario, for example, is just tired, Jasmine is almost constantly wired, and Tracy is tired *and* wired. Their different symptoms reflect the various ways in which chronic stress has affected both their HPA axes and the rest of their bodies' systems, which are in constant communication.

However different their symptoms, though, all three women have one thing in common: the long-term exposure to *chronic stress*. Excessive unrelenting stress has profoundly affected each woman's emotions, mind, and spirit as well as her body. One significant result of chronic stress is an ever-increasing *allostatic load*.

The concept of allostatic load was coined in 1993 by researchers Bruce McEwen and Eliot Stellar to express the profound and ongoing ways that stress affects the body and all its systems. We're used to thinking of stress as "just" stress—an annoying problem to shake off, or a habit of feeling worried or anxious. But from a medical point of view, long-term chronic stress has an enormous and very real impact on the body. The stress our body bears—our allostatic load—is a burden that affects our heart and our brain, as well as our circulatory, nervous, endocrine, digestive, and immune systems.

Each of us was born with a unique genetic makeup, and each of us has lived a different history. These differences are written into our bodies, giving each of us our own roster of strengths and weaknesses. So when our allostatic load begins to increase, we each respond differently. Some of us get headaches, others develop backaches. Some of us get depressed, others become anxious. Some of us may develop high blood pressure, while others find that our blood pressure is too low. We might develop insomnia—or perhaps we'll sleep more than usual and feel foggy and tired even when awake. Our symptoms will vary, but they all reveal the same underlying problem: we are staggering under the burden of our allostatic load. (For information on how to check your allostatic load, see Appendix B.)

Often, women with adrenal dysfunction have experienced extraordinary stress in their childhoods, their adult lives, or both. They may have been beaten or sexually abused as children, or they may have been expected to take care of a parent, or younger brothers and sisters while a parent was unavailable. As adults, they may have had to raise a child with serious behavior problems, cope with a child's chronic disease, or deal with aging parents. Alternatively, they may only have experienced moderate stress in childhood and/or adulthood, but over time, the stress accumulates. In some cases their coping skills simply wear out; in others, they weren't taught sufficient coping skills to begin with. Either way, their stress-induced allostatic load is creating adrenal dysfunction.

The "Wired" Racehorse

The Racehorse is one of three basic adrenal profiles I identified in Chapter 1. Though these aren't hard-and-fast medical diagnoses, they do help us understand the way in which physical and emotional symptoms tend to cluster together.

The biology behind the Racehorse is simple: she's responding to a chronic flow of stress hormones, living in a near-constant adrenaline rush. Her system is coursing with adrenaline (a.k.a. epinephrine), noradrenaline (a.k.a. norepinephrine), and cortisol, which keep her heart pounding, her blood pumping, her pupils dilated, and her nerves on edge. Her adrenals are also providing her system with high levels of DHEA, the "mother hormone," so called because it is one of the key precursors for many of the other hormones that contribute to energy and a sense of well-being as well as many of the hormonal biological effects in our bodies.

Yet sometimes patients of this type are surprised when I share their lab results with them. Although the stress hormones would seem to create a constant state of energy and feeling "wired," they'll often look at me and say, "But I'm just so tired!" Although her system is racing, the Racehorse may feel exhausted—eloquent testimony to the fact that we can only burn that hot and that fast for so long without a counterreaction.

As we've seen, we rely upon both our *sympathetic nervous system,* which revs us up, and our *parasympathetic nervous system,* which calms us down. Specifically, the sympathetic nervous system uses such hormones as cortisol and DHEA to prepare us for exertion. Then, when exertion is no longer needed, the parasympathetic nervous system uses "anti-stress" biochemicals, such as acetylcholine (ACh) and nitrous oxide (NO), to reverse that "revving up" process and help to calm us down.

In particular, the parasympathetic reaction needs to reverse the elements of the fight-or-flight reaction. The sympathetic nervous system gets our heart beating faster and our blood pumping harder; the parasympathetic nervous system encourages our heartbeat to slow and our blood pressure to return to normal. The sympathetic nervous system widens our pupils so we can see danger coming; the parasympathetic nervous system encourages our pupils to constrict so we don't have to remain so alert and anxious. Our sympathetic nervous system sends blood flowing to our muscles so we can run; our parasympathetic nervous system sends it back to our intestines so we can digest our food. Our sympathetic nervous system causes our stomach to contract and encourages our colon to eliminate waste quickly; our parasympathetic nervous system returns our gastrointestinal tract to its normal relaxed state so it can do an optimal job of digestion and elimination.

When a too-active sympathetic nervous system—via a too-constant production of stress hormones—prevents this soothing parasympathetic reaction, we eventually feel tired and worn out, even as our levels of stress hormones remain high. Yet no matter how tired we are, the cortisol and DHEA also cause us to feel wired.

Because there is so much cross talk between the HPA axis and the body's other systems, the Racehorse is likely to suffer from a wide variety of symptoms, which will, like Jasmine's, almost certainly worsen as she gets older. Her thyroid function may be *down-regulated,* which means that it's not working up to its full potential and not producing enough T4, which converts to T3 (two key types of thyroid hormone). Since thyroid is used by every cell in the body to regulate its metabolism, low levels of thyroid can create numerous problems, including weight gain, fatigue, and depression.

Like the adrenals, the thyroid gland is at the end of a chain of command that starts with the hypothalamus and passes through the pituitary. Just as chronic stress affects the HPA axis, it also affects the HPT (hypothalamic-pituitary-thyroid) axis as well. Because of the enormous amount of cross talk that goes on along these axes, thyroid problems can be triggered by adrenal problems and can often be cleared up when the adrenals are brought back into balance.

Another potential problem the Racehorse faces is Hashimoto's thyroiditis, an auto-immune condition that causes the body's immune system to mistake the thyroid hor-mone for a foreign agent and to progressively destroy the thyroid tissues. As a result, the thyroid attempts to compensate for the amount that is being destroyed, often by prolif-erating new thyroid follicles. In this case, two of the Racehorse's glands are overworking, and both are at risk for becoming exhausted. Fortunately, healing the adrenals may go a long way toward lifting the burden on the thyroid.

The Racehorse is also at risk for mild gastrointestinal disturbances, since the chronic stress hormones are interfering with her stomach's ability to digest and her colon's abili-ty to eliminate waste. In order for the stomach and the colon to work properly, they need signals from both the revving-up sympathetic nervous system and the calming-down parasympathetic nervous system. The Racehorse is mainly getting only the revving-up signal, however, which throws her digestion out of balance.

The wired Racehorse keeps herself "up" almost all the time, with no chance for the parasympathetic nervous system to kick in. As a result, she's wearing herself down, with-out even realizing it. If she ever sits quietly for a few minutes—perhaps in the waiting room of a doctor's office where she's not allowed to use her cell phone or can't get recep-tion for it—she suddenly falls asleep. When she wakes, though, even from a longer sleep, she almost never feels well rested. The stress-hormone levels in her blood are still too high.

As we have also seen, the stress reaction mobilizes aldosterone, which regulates fluid retention and electrolyte balance. When cortisol levels are too high for too long, they set off a biochemical chain of events that shuts down the aldosterone production. As a result, the Racehorse may suffer from low blood pressure, bloating, and perhaps also a craving for salt, which she needs to balance her electrolytes.

Often, the Racehorse doesn't feel hungry—again, those stress hormones were designed to kill the appetite until the fight-or-flight emergency is over. Just as she suddenly finds herself nodding off, however, she may find herself suddenly ravenous—or hungry all the time. Both her fluctuating energy levels and her rapidly changing hunger are symp-toms of dysregulated blood sugar, which also lead her to be tempted by sweets and starchy foods that will quickly boost her energy back up to the wired state she's grown accustomed to—only to "crash" once more when the effect of the sugars and the simple carbs wears off.

The Racehorse is rarely interested in sex, either, and often can't fully enjoy it even when she does have it. That's because of the cross talk between the HPA axis and the hormonal system. Our estrogen and progesterone are made primarily in the ovaries until perimenopause and menopause, when the adrenals help to compensate for the ovaries' shutting down by producing small amounts of sex hormones. After menopause, the adrenals are our main source of testosterone, too, which is crucial to our libido and drive.

So there are a few different ways that disturbances of the HPA axis can affect our sexual feelings and responses, as well as our menstrual and premenstrual experience. First, nature designed the fight-or-flight reaction to focus on immediate survival. Long-term considerations, such as digestion and reproduction, are far less important when your life is in danger. As a result, stress kills our appetite, interferes with digestion, and shuts down our sex drive—and can shut down our fertility, too. If the soothing parasympathetic response doesn't come often enough or fully enough, we may end up with ongoing problems in all these areas.

When cortisol levels remain high and never fall as they are intended to, they can create significant imbalances in our sex hormones. Too much stress can also interfere with our menstrual cycle, perimenopause, and menopause. Once again, an imbalance between our sympathetic and parasympathetic nervous systems has played havoc with our lives.

Years ago, I saw an article in a magazine for pregnant women about women who had undergone "amazing experiences" while they were expecting. One woman ran a marathon despite having a fractured ankle. Another woman who was nine months pregnant and having contractions hiked to the top of a mountain. Although the article presented these women as modern heroines, I was appalled. Why are we pushing ourselves to such extremes? Our bodies understand these demands as extraordinary states of emergency. They hunker down, hold on to fat, and shut down every system we don't need. As a result, the Racehorse has begun to gain weight, to have trouble digesting her food, and to lose her sex drive.

The constant stress of the Racehorse's life may also lead to headaches, tension in the neck, or back pain. She's probably been told by lots of people to "lighten up" or "take it easy once in a while," but as one Racehorse patient told me, "If I ever did sit down, I'd feel like I could never get up again."

Those high levels of stress hormones often create a constant state of anxiety, which in turn interferes with memory and concentration. The Racehorse's racing heart may develop palpitations. And while the stress hormones usually keep blood away from the skin (in case of injury during fight or flight), a temporary "crash" may cause flushing and redness.

Despite the downsides, the Racehorse often enjoys her adrenaline rush, and she may work in a profession that relies on this type of high-octane performance. Emergency-room staff and other medical professionals, police officers, firefighters, small-business owners, journalists on tight deadlines, freelance writers and artists, lawyers who deal with high-pressure workloads, and financial professionals like Jasmine may spend a significant portion of their workday coping with emergencies or struggling to do the impossible—over and over and over again. They may thrive in the high-stress atmosphere and even develop a kind of addiction to it, feeling that anything less charged with intensity and danger is, well, kind of boring.

I think also of the poignant story told in the Academy Award–winning movie *The Hurt Locker,* in which a combat veteran just can't adjust to the mundane chores of civilian life. By the film's last scene, he's back on the front lines, risking his life as he tries to disarm yet another bomb. There's even an epigraph from former *New York Times* war correspondent Chris Hedges that sums up this point: "The rush of battle is often a potent and lethal addiction, for war is a drug." The soldier might not have been a Racehorse by nature, but he had surely become one under fire.

Much as the Racehorse may enjoy her high-performance life, she can get worn down by it. Sometimes she might feel on the verge of unbelievable irritation or feel hyper, strung out, or as though she simply can't tolerate even the smallest irritation. She may overreact to tiny problems and then feel deep regret, not understanding why she lost her temper or was suddenly filled with despair.

A multitasker with apparently boundless energy, the Racehorse may suddenly feel at a loss whenever she has to stop. Moments of quiet are when everything catches up with her, whether it's the anxiety over all she has to do or the fears and sorrows from her childhood that she may be keeping at bay with her frantic pace. Her parents may have inadvertently given her the message that no matter how much she does, it's not enough, or she may be reacting to some difficulty her folks had during her childhood, which she still feels bad about not being able to fix. The pain of these experiences, which feel to her like failures, may overwhelm her in quiet moments or down times, even if she's not aware of why she feels so angry with herself or so depressed.

Remember, the amygdala carries a strong emotional charge from key events in our lives, but our conscious mind doesn't necessarily remember things the same way. Our feelings seem to take on a life of their own, and the Racehorse's feelings may bubble up whenever she isn't busy. When she sleeps, she may grind her teeth, a sign of the anger or the tension she carries within her that doesn't always have an outlet in her waking life. Or she may have developed a nervous habit, such as biting her nails.

The Racehorse might have a tendency to be rigid with herself, perhaps as the adults she knew while growing up were rigid with her. She may push herself to exercise hard, even when she starts to feel tired rather than energized. As the effects of the cortisol start to take their toll, she'll find herself gaining weight around the middle, no matter how strictly she diets or how vigorously she exercises. This can be extremely frustrating, because she has such high expectations for herself and becomes so disappointed when she doesn't meet them. If the Racehorse has children, she expects herself to be a good mother, and is often discouraged by how far short she falls—in her opinion, at least—of the marks she sets for herself. If other people praise her, thank her, or suggest that she's too hard on herself and that she has accomplished more than she realizes, she may respond politely, but inside she feels despair. Don't they understand how little she's getting done? Don't they realize how much more she has to do?

Often the women I treat of this type are somewhat impatient. They may be fidgety and have a hard time sitting still. They may be particularly impatient when it comes to their own feelings. "I don't have time to deal with all these emotions!" one patient told me when I gently suggested that she look at some of the sources for the stress in her life.

"Look, what's done is done," another woman told me when I tried to relate her extreme self-criticism to her highly critical—and wounded—mother. "I don't believe in digging up the past—I believe in living in the present!" Living in the present is an excellent motto, but unfortunately, my self-critical patient actually *was* living in the past. Anytime she failed to live up to her extraordinarily high expectation of herself, she scolded herself exactly as her mother had scolded her, not realizing that her mother, too, had suffered from her own bouts of self-hatred and despair. Although she wasn't consciously aware that her dissatisfaction with herself came from her mother, her amygdala was still triggered by any situation that didn't work out perfectly—situations that had, during her childhood, set her mother off.

The Racehorse can be an extraordinary person to have in your corner if you need someone to accomplish the impossible for you. She never gives up, and she has enormous willpower and drive. Her challenge is to allow herself some downtime, to come to terms with her emotional baggage—we all have some!—and to give her parasympathetic nervous system a chance to counterbalance the stimulating effect of her adrenals.

The Tired and Wired Workhorse

I've identified a second adrenal profile that I call the Workhorse. Again, this isn't a firm medical diagnosis, but it is a useful way to recognize a common form of adrenal dysfunction. The Workhorse has many of the same symptoms as the Racehorse, but she also has another set of symptoms that seem to contradict them. That's because sometimes her body is surging with stress hormones, creating that wired feeling, while at other times, her body is feeling the first signs of adrenal fatigue, as her adrenals occasionally underproduce.

The Workhorse, in particular, experiences a 24-hour cycle that is out of whack. As we've seen in previous chapters, our cortisol levels are supposed to peak in the morning, helping us to wake up energized and ready for the challenges of the day. They fluctuate somewhat as the day wears on, but generally, they begin to drop as night falls, so that we can relax into a restful sleep.

The Workhorse, by contrast, is tired in the morning, since her adrenals haven't quite kicked into gear. She might start her day with two, three, even five cups of coffee, but no matter how many artificial stimulants she takes, she finds herself dragging through the morning. She might have a bit more energy in midmorning and then crash after lunch, as the need to digest her food invokes the parasympathetic nervous system, which also induces her to relax. Or she might remain low until the afternoon and then steadily gain energy into the evening. Another possibility is that she stays low through the afternoon and wishes she could take a nap after lunch. Either way, by nighttime, her HPA axis is signaling her adrenals for a fresh supply of cortisol and suddenly she's totally wired, often feeling anxious as well. *What's wrong with me?* she wonders. *Why can't I get on the same schedule as other people?*

By evening, the Workhorse's stress levels are peaking, a combination of the caffeine she's been mainlining and the stress that's been building over the day. Her stress-hormone levels are high, and now she'll be wide awake for hours. Or perhaps she'll fall into an exhausted sleep only to wake at 2 A.M., her heart pounding, her thoughts racing. Although at least some of her late-night anxiety is fueled by sugar and caffeine, it feels to the Workhorse as though she's simply overwhelmed by real-life concerns. *What if my boss gets mad at me? What if something goes wrong with the kids? What if I can't pay my bills? What if Joel never calls back and I never have another boyfriend?* These fears multiply and intensify and seem all too real, as the possibility of sleep recedes further and further.

Some of the Workhorse's sleep problems have to do with caffeine. If she's been mainlining it all day, there will be enough in her system by nightfall to keep her from falling or staying asleep.

Some of the sleep problems may come from a blood-sugar imbalance. The Workhorse often uses sugary or starchy foods to restore her flagging energy. She likes the quick burst of energy they give her, since they're metabolized so quickly, raising her blood-sugar levels. Eventually, though, the Workhorse feels a sugar crash, and so again she turns to sweets and starches, along with her beloved caffeine. As a result, her blood sugar is out of balance, which can interfere with sleep patterns.

An even bigger portion of the problem, though, goes back to the lack of balance between the sympathetic and the parasympathetic nervous systems. All day long, the Workhorse is coping with high levels of stress, and she's constantly trying to rev herself up to cope with them—through sugar and caffeine, yes, but also in her attitude and behavior. Then, at night, she's wired, still in hypersympathetic mode. Because she hasn't done anything to get into "parasympathetic mode," her body doesn't know it's supposed to relax.

Often a Workhorse keeps herself in sympathetic mode well into the evening. Right up until she goes to bed, she may be doing household chores, working on her computer, or thinking hard about the problems she has to solve. Her body never gets the signals: *Calm down. Relax. Slow your heartbeat. Slow your breathing. Stop flooding your system with stress hormones and start filling it with relaxation hormones.* Sleep is far more difficult as a result.

If the Workhorse uses a computer or even watches television before bed, that can compound the sleep problem. The flickering light of the electronic screen actually signals the brain to *wake up.* That's why people with sleep problems are advised to avoid all electronic screens for at least an hour before bedtime. (We'll talk more about ways to overcome sleep problems in Chapter 7.)

So here we have the makings of a truly vicious cycle. Not sleeping causes the Workhorse to feel tired throughout the day, fatigue leads her to rely on caffeine, and caffeine prevents her from sleeping, causing her to feel even more tired.

There's also a kind of feedback loop between insomnia and anxiety—the less able you are to sleep, the more anxious you feel; the more anxious you feel, the less able you are to sleep. The anxiety further prevents the Workhorse from getting into parasympathetic mode: when you fear danger, you can't signal your body to give up its defenses, and of course, sleep is the most defenseless state of all. So the Workhorse is often caught in a seemingly endless spiral of anxiety, sleeplessness, and fatigue.

The fatigue leads to another type of downward spiral. Because the Workhorse is so often exhausted, she begins to give up on activities that she once enjoyed. She becomes increasingly isolated, even reclusive. Partly as a result of these life circumstances and partly due to the biochemical effects of chronic stress, she often falls prey to depression, feeling hopeless, helpless, listless, and despairing—first only occasionally, then more often.

The stress takes its toll on the Workhorse's body as well as her brain. Her hair may begin to thin, or she may lose her body hair. Her blood pressure may drop, causing her to feel dizzy when she gets up in the morning or to feel faint if she stands up too quickly. This is as a result of low aldosterone production, which may also cause her to crave salt.

Since there is so much cross talk between the HPA axis and the gut, adrenal dysfunction can create digestive disorders, causing the Workhorse to suffer from diarrhea, constipation, or abdominal pain. As we have seen, the sympathetic and the parasympathetic nervous systems must be working in tandem for the stomach and colon to operate properly. If the sympathetic nervous system is working overtime (and becoming fatigued), while the parasympathetic nervous system isn't working enough, our entire gastrointestinal system is at risk.

Like the Racehorse, the Workhorse may be vulnerable to thyroid problems, since the HPA axis communicates so closely with the thyroid. Since chronic stress weakens the immune system, she may suddenly be getting more infections, or, like Tracy the social worker, be sick all winter. She may also feel increasingly sensitive to changes in the weather or develop an increasing sensitivity to environmental toxins.

Like the Racehorse, the Workhorse may also feel an increased sensitivity to life stress, becoming irritable for no apparent reason or bursting into tears at the slightest setback. She may be especially on edge with her children or loved ones, partly because she wants so much to come through for them, and, with her increasing fatigue, feels so frustrated that she can't.

Just as her physical symptoms are somewhat contradictory, the Workhorse might experience contradictory psychological symptoms, too. She may feel wired and anxious some of the time, while at other times she feels as though she has no drive or motivation. She may be angry with herself for just dragging through the daylight hours, or she might feel mildly depressed, wondering, *What's the point?* One patient who fit this profile told me plaintively, "I used to be such a good multitasker, but now I can barely get one thing done in an entire day. I used to bounce back quickly over the weekend and have some time for fun with my boyfriend, but now I'm just exhausted on Friday night and I barely feel like myself even by Sunday."

The Workhorse's real frustrations come out when anyone suggests she take better care of herself. "I don't have *time* to shop and cook all those healthy meals, and I don't like to cook anyway," one woman told me. "All your suggestions sound really good in theory, but I just don't have the energy to do any of them."

As with the Racehorse, I hear echoes of angry, frustrated, and depressed parents whenever my Workhorse patients criticize themselves. I can imagine the little girl being told that Mommy is disappointed in her. I can see the bewildered teenager coping with a mother who sometimes wanted lots of attention and sometimes simply wanted to be left alone. While I believe that all parents do the best they can, and that parents who fall short are simply struggling with the legacy of their own imperfect parents, I can also see how deeply a parent's words can cut and how lasting a mark their attitudes can leave. When a patient tells me that she just isn't "very disciplined" or "can't seem to find the energy" to take care of herself, or doesn't think she'll "be able to say 'no'" to one more demand at home or at work, I can see the child whose parents never managed to communicate to her how valuable she was, what a delight it was to take care of her, what a pleasure she was to be with. I see a child whose parents conveyed—without ever meaning to or wanting to—that she was a burden to care for and a disappointment to be around. And so I see a grown woman sitting in my office, letting me know that taking care of herself feels like a burden, she can never make time for it—and she doesn't understand why.

The Workhorse has remarkable resources to offer, and she's willing to put her head down and soldier through for her co-workers, her boss, her community, and her family. She'll offer her mind, her heart, and her spirit in the service of what she believes in, and she won't allow herself to stop until the job is done. Her challenges are to allow herself some comfort and support; to take a look at the historical sources of her stress; and to begin the adrenal-friendly regimen of calming foods, herbal supplements, and self-care that could heal her adrenal imbalance.

The Tired Flatliner

The third adrenal profile I've identified is the Flatliner. This woman is tired. Bone tired. Although she doesn't test positive for Addison's disease, she has some of the same symptoms as a person with the condition's full-scale adrenal burnout. She's so exhausted, she might even have to take frequent rests while preparing dinner or playing with her children. And when the weekend comes, she can barely conceive of getting up and dressed, let alone leaving the house.

Over the years, high cortisol levels have interfered with the Flatliner's production of aldosterone, which we rely on to prevent fluid retention and maintain electrolyte balance. As a result, the Flatliner often struggles with low blood pressure, feeling dizzy when she wakes up and craving salt all the time. In the morning, she craves sugar, too, relying on sweet, starchy foods to get her going. Like the Workhorse, the Flatliner may be losing hair, on her head or on her body.

The Flatliner has been struggling for a long time under a heavy allostatic load. Her stress certainly has its emotional roots, but she may be also suffering from one or more physical stressors, such as environmental sensitivity or some kind of chronic pain, infection, or illness that has further taxed her adrenals and stressed her entire system as well.

As a result, the Flatliner often faces some type of thyroid disorder. Her allostatic load may have become so heavy that she also has developed an autoimmune condition (asthma, rheumatoid arthritis, lupus, antiphospholipid syndrome), a gastrointestinal problem, a cardiovascular disorder, or perhaps several conditions at once. These disorders put further stress on her HPA axis and on her body's other systems, creating still more strain for her exhausted adrenals. As a result, they can no longer produce stress hormones in the quantities she needs to feel happy and energized.

Weight gain can be a symptom for all types of adrenal dysfunction, but it's particularly challenging for the Flatliner. Her system has long since come to believe it's in the state of chronic emergency described in Chapter 2, in which every bit of body fat must be maintained, regardless of diet or exercise. Think of our ancestors trekking across the desert—what would have happened to them if eating less and exercising more had burned off *their* body fat? They would have withered away to nothing! The Flatliner's body believes it's facing a similar crisis, and so it holds on to excess weight that is itself creating health problems.

The Flatliner may also be suffering from insulin resistance, a condition that promotes weight gain. (I'll explain insulin resistance in more detail in Chapter 5.) If she's overweight, the excess fat is producing a lot of cytokines, which promote inflammation. Years of sustained high cortisol production have led to the high levels of glucocorticoids that promote inflammation. As we saw in Chapter 2, acute inflammation is the body's healing response to infection or injury—but too much inflammation can cause problems of its own. As a result, the Flatliner is at great risk of heart disease, diabetes, cancer, and autoimmune conditions such as allergies, asthma, rheumatoid arthritis, and many others.

The Flatliner may be depressed, both because of her life circumstances (her health problems, her overwhelming responsibilities, the lack of energy that limits her activities) and because of her hormonal imbalance. The accumulated stress of the last several years—perhaps the last several decades—has almost certainly worn her down. She may have a hard time leaving the house if she doesn't have to. She can't imagine having to cope with one more thing. The tiniest problem becomes a disaster. The tiniest task becomes an enormous chore. From her point of view, her emotional resources are worn almost to the bone, and she just doesn't have anything left—to enjoy herself, to enjoy her partner or her kids, to cope with even one more challenge, however small. Now, in her 50s or 60s, as menopause takes over, she feels as though she is beginning to collapse under the burden of all those years devoted to others.

The Flatliner may be more sensitive to stress, collapsing under an allostatic load that another woman might have been able to bear. We don't really know all the factors that go into making one woman more vulnerable to stress than another, but I suspect it has something to do with how well you listen to your body. If your response to being tired is to stop, turn off the phone, and take a nap, or to build restful, pleasurable days off into your schedule, or even to take a ten-minute break when you truly relax, you may be able to cope with greater burdens than if you simply soldier on, pushing yourself harder and harder without relief.

Sometimes when my Flatliner patients speak to me, I hear the desperate efforts of a little girl trying to rise above the abuse or neglect or mixed messages generated by her own parents' pain. I see the confused teenager trying to sort out why some people seem to have such fortunate lives and others seem to have it so hard. I can only imagine the fortitude it takes for her to believe even a little bit that someday things might get better.

At other times, I hear the child who has an apparently happy childhood, but whose mother and father rarely gave themselves a break, rarely allowed themselves to enjoy their lives, perhaps because they were immigrants wanting to prove themselves or people whose families lost it all during the Great Depression and spent the rest of their lives trying to make up for it. I see the teenage girl trying obediently to please other people, to take care of her family, to rise to the occasion even when she might prefer to be "selfish" or "bad."

The Flatliner has shown amazing courage in the face of a series of blows or demands. She has been resilient, resourceful, and valiant in coping with her life's challenges as she continues to come through for others, again and again and again. She has the capacity to make one more set of changes—to change her diet, lifestyle, and relationship to stress so that she can finally heal her adrenals—but she doesn't always believe in herself enough to try. Her challenge is to own the struggle she has waged all her life and choose now to lay down some of the burden of her allostatic load.

Toxic Responsiveness

For all three adrenal types, the stress experienced by their HPA axis may translate to a suppression of the immune system, causing them to be ultrasensitive to any stressor in their environment: noise; changes in the weather; and toxins in their food, cosmetics, homes, or community. All three adrenal types may also find themselves hypersensitive to even tiny changes in their environments or their lives, since the adrenal reserves that they would ordinarily use to cope with change simply aren't there. They've been used up by the constant influx of stress hormones from the chronic experience of stress.

Adrenal healing can often ease the pain of toxic responsiveness. As your adrenal reserves are restored, you may find yourself newly able to tolerate things that once made you feel ill and to handle life's challenges with a calm and confidence that you haven't known in years—or maybe have never known. Start making little changes now and eventually, they may lead to large and lasting changes in your health, energy, and sense of well-being.

ADRENAL-FRIENDLY ACTIVITIES: WAYS TO BEGIN TO HEAL

- *Journal about change.* Give yourself from 5 minutes to 30 minutes and complete all or part of the following journaling exercise. Answer as quickly and spontaneously as you can, writing as much or as little as you like without stopping to think.

  1. If I could change one thing about my life right now, it would be _____.

  2. I would like to change it because _____.

  3. What I would do differently is _____.

  4. When I imagine that the entire change has been made in the best possible way, what I imagine is _____.

  5. If I were to make that change, my first step might be to _____.

- *Visualize a conversation about change.* Take 5 to 10 minutes to complete the following visualization. If you like, pick up your journal afterward and write for a few minutes about the experience and what it meant to you:

> *You are entering a beautiful but very thick green forest, following a path that winds through the bushes and trees. After walking for a few minutes, you come to a clearing, and there waiting for you is a powerful being who can give you all the help you need and answer any question you have. This can be someone you know, someone you've heard of, or a creature you are simply imagining. Walk into the clearing and have a conversation with this being. Say or ask anything you want and listen to the answers. Then, when you're ready, thank the being, turn around, and return through the woods until you've come back out again. Carry with you whatever you learned from your conversation.*

- *Relax into sleep.* The key to falling asleep is not to think about sleep itself but to allow your mind to focus on a relaxing activity. One option is to focus your mind on relaxing your body—not with the goal of sleeping but with the goal of enjoying the experience of lying in bed.

  Begin with your toes. Allow them to enjoy the feel of the sheets and blankets, the warmth of your bed, the relief of not having to support your body. Move down to your heels. What do you notice as they press into your soft, firm mattress? How do your feet feel without your whole weight on them? Move up to your shins and your calves. Notice the softness of the sheets against them and the pleasant weight of the blankets. Notice their exact temperature—are they cool or warm?

  Continue in that way until you've reached the crown of your head. You will either fall asleep during or soon after the exercise, or you will have done something enjoyable for a few minutes. If you don't feel drowsy, turn on the light and read until you do—but no computer or television. The flickering light in the electronic screen will stimulate you and keep you awake.

Healing Your Adrenal Type

Although I've identified three adrenal types, I'm very much aware that every woman has her own story. However, I encourage you to choose the adrenal type that seems to fit your condition most closely, as the kinds of herbs and supplements I recommend in Chapter 5, and the type of exercise I suggest in Chapter 7, will be based on your adrenal type. The wired Racehorse needs a regimen very different from the exhausted Flatliner—and the tired and wired Workhorse needs a program tailored to her own specific symptoms.

Meanwhile, what else can you do to heal? Whatever your adrenal type, I suggest you give yourself time to be quiet and consider what you want deep in your heart. All too often, the life you want looks quite different from the life you currently have.

Once you have spent time reflecting, consider taking some steps to make your vision come true. You might be looking at little steps—taking a few minutes each day to breathe, buying flowers for an "adult" dinner with your partner or friends as you let the kids eat first, saying "no" to your boss or your friend or your mother-in-law. Or you might be looking at bigger changes: enrolling in a yoga class, making new, healthier food choices, turning off the computer by dinnertime or leaving it off all weekend, changing a relationship or a job or a career plan.

Whatever you decide and however big or small your steps, I urge you to be patient with yourself, gentle with yourself, and committed to yourself. The danger that looms ahead is a progression into worse symptoms, more severe problems, and a more despairing frame of mind. The promise that looms even larger is the opportunity to heal yourself, restore your energy, and regain your joy—to feel like yourself again. I believe you're worth whatever effort it takes to make that happen—and I hope you do, too.

THE THREE DEGREES OF ADRENAL DYSFUNCTION

As we have seen, adrenal dysfunction is a progressive disease. It tends to start with small symptoms that are easy to ignore or attribute to other causes. Left unaddressed, it gradually progresses to symptoms that are both more numerous and more severe.

If you can catch adrenal dysfunction when the symptoms are still mild, you'll be ahead of the game, because that's when it's easiest to reverse the condition. If your symptoms have progressed to "moderate" or "severe," you'll probably need longer to heal, though you absolutely can do it.

As you move forward with Part II, you'll need to figure out how severe your adrenal dysfunction has become. That's because the treatments vary to some extent, depending on how far along you are:

- When your symptoms are still mild, your adrenal glands are producing stress hormones too often, with little or no downtime for your parasympathetic nervous system to bring relaxation and balance. This is the phase in which you most often feel "wired."

- In the moderate phase of adrenal dysfunction, your adrenal glands are still flooding your body with stress hormones, but they're beginning to get depleted, so you feel both tired and wired.

- In the severe phase, your adrenal glands are completely depleted—and so are you. This is when you feel as though your get-up-and-go has gotten up and gone. Mainly you just feel tired.

Whatever stage your adrenal dysfunction has reached, it's important for you to identify it and take steps to rebalance and heal. Catching adrenal dysfunction when it's still in the *mild* phase is ideal, because you can spare yourself months or even years of fatigue, irritability, sleep disturbances, and excess weight. But even if you become aware of the problem by the *moderate* or *severe* phase, you can still turn the situation around. It just may take a little longer for your body to restore itself. Just honor yourself enough to take the steps to get better.

The first order of business is to find out exactly what you have to deal with. Start by taking the following questionnaire to figure out where you are along the adrenal spectrum.

Where Are You on the Adrenal Spectrum?

Identify any symptom you've experienced in the last three months. Here's how to score your symptoms:

- *Mild:* A minor issue—it doesn't affect me much.

- *Moderate:* A real problem, but I push myself through it.

- *Severe:* I can barely function or deal with it.

	None	Mild	Moderate	Severe
1. I have difficulty falling asleep.	○	○	○	○
2. I have difficulty staying asleep.	○	○	○	○
3. I feel very tired, especially in the afternoon, or after lunch between 2 P.M. and 3 P.M.	○	○	○	○
4. I am exhausted in the morning, or I feel "bone tired" when I wake up.	○	○	○	○
5. I am fatigued all the time and have little stamina.	○	○	○	○
6. I feel that I've gained weight in the last year, especially around my middle, and I don't understand why.	○	○	○	○
7. I lose my temper easily, or I am irritable or depressed— and I should know better!	○	○	○	○
8. I have thinning hair or eyebrows, or I suffer from hair loss.	○	○	○	○
9. I have acne.	○	○	○	○
10. I regularly use caffeinated beverages such as coffee or soda to jump-start me or get me through the day.	○	○	○	○
11. I am forgetful, fuzzy-minded, or absentminded.	○	○	○	○
12. I crave sweets, carbohydrates, or sugar.	○	○	○	○
13. I crave salt.	○	○	○	○
14. I have frequent infections.	○	○	○	○
15. I am intolerant to cold weather or temperature changes.	○	○	○	○
16. The smallest thing sets me off.	○	○	○	○

	None	Mild	Moderate	Severe
17. My zest for life has waned— my get-up-and-go has gotten up and gone!	○	○	○	○
18. I feel faint if I get up too quickly.	○	○	○	○
19. I find myself falling asleep while watching TV, a movie, or a play.	○	○	○	○
20. I never seem to be able to finish reading a book because I'm always falling asleep.	○	○	○	○
21. I feel exhausted after dealing with anything stressful.	○	○	○	○
22. I feel drained rather than energized after I exercise.	○	○	○	○
23. I often run out of energy during the day.	○	○	○	○
24. I feel shaky if I don't eat regularly.	○	○	○	○
25. I perk up at 9 P.M. after being tired throughout the day.	○	○	○	○
26. I often use high-fat foods to get more energy.	○	○	○	○
27. I crave high-protein, high-fat, salty foods like meats and cheeses.	○	○	○	○
28. I crave sweets—they help my energy.	○	○	○	○
29. I feel somewhat unwell most of the time.	○	○	○	○
30. I often have low blood pressure.	○	○	○	○
31. I have periodic episodes of total body weakness.	○	○	○	○
32. I am deeply affected by severe weather changes.	○	○	○	○
33. My productivity at work has decreased.	○	○	○	○
34. My anxiety level has markedly increased.	○	○	○	○

Now add up your symptoms. Give yourself 1 point for "mild," 2 points for "moderate," and 3 points for "severe." Here's how to interpret your score:

- *0–8 points:* Congratulations. You have effectively prevented adrenal dysfunction and are enjoying good hormonal health. To continue your good health, see the diet, exercise, lifestyle, and emotional reprogramming suggestions in Part II.

- *9–17 points:* You are experiencing mild adrenal dysfunction. You have probably been able to dismiss your symptoms or attribute them to some other cause. Now that you have correctly identified them as adrenal dysfunction, you can use the suggestions in Part II to turn the situation around and restore your adrenal health.

- *18–25 points:* You are struggling with moderate adrenal dysfunction. Your daily life is seriously affected by your symptoms and you may be actively looking for solutions. The suggestions in Part II can make a substantial difference in restoring your adrenal health.

- *26 points or more:* You are suffering from severe adrenal dysfunction. While you may need to stick with the suggestions in Part II for two or three months, you will be able to see a significant improvement within 30 days.

Know Where You're Headed

When patients come to me with severe symptoms, they're keenly aware that they have a problem—indeed, many of them have already been to two or three other practitioners who were unable to help. But when patients come in with mild symptoms—a little extra weight, some unexplained fatigue—they're often surprised to hear that these relatively minor issues are actually the signs of potentially greater problems to come.

When you see the body as an integrated whole, however, you recognize both that these minor problems add up, and that they are all indicators of a disturbing trend. I never want to alarm my patients (or my readers), but I do want you to understand that even if you just have *mild* symptoms of adrenal dysfunction, you may be headed down a road you won't like—and you may be farther along than you think. Mild symptoms now can be the signs of more serious problems later on, especially if you run into a major stressor, such as the loss of a job, a divorce, a move to another community, or a family member's serious illness. Suddenly that addition to your allostatic load becomes the straw that broke the camel's back, and minor ailments turn into major concerns.

This is not a cue to become alarmed, but it is a plea to pay attention. No matter what challenges you're facing or how busy you are, consider finding ways—even little ones—to soothe and comfort yourself, release your stress, and let your parasympathetic nervous system bring your body back into balance.

Addicted to Busyness?

My patient Cheryl was by anyone's standards an accomplished woman. Although her parents had barely made it through high school and struggled to keep a roof over their heads, Cheryl had somehow managed to put herself through college and law school and had become a successful lawyer. By day she worked for a corporate law firm in Boston, but she decided that life was healthier in southern Maine, so she managed to commute 90 minutes each way so that her children could grow up in what she considered a nicer area. She also thought it was important to give back to the community, so in her "spare time" she volunteered her legal services to a local environmental group, a community-action group, and a few other worthy organizations. She and her husband had three children, all of whom attended private school, so Cheryl had huge bills to pay, as well as a share in the fund-raising responsibilities that every parent was supposed to take part in.

When Cheryl began having symptoms of adrenal dysfunction, she found no relief from the first three practitioners she visited. By the time she came to see me, she was in her late 30s and had *moderate* symptoms of adrenal dysfunction: tired and wired, she was sleeping poorly; dragging herself through the day; and felt anxious, depressed, and overwhelmed. She confessed that she'd started snapping at the children lately, even when she knew they were trying to be nice, and that sometimes at work it was all she could do to keep from bursting into tears. "I'm just so *busy*," she kept repeating. "It just never *stops.*"

But when I tried to explore with her where in her busy life she might cut back and do a bit less, Cheryl balked repeatedly. "I can't give up *that,*" she replied at every suggestion I made. "I have to do it. Everyone is counting on me. You don't understand—I'm the only one who can do it; if I don't, everything falls apart. My children need me, my husband needs me, my community needs me—everybody needs me. There isn't a single thing I'm doing that I feel I could give up."

Finally, I said to her point-blank, "Cheryl, maybe you like being busy."

Cheryl stared at me, on the verge of tears. "I *don't*. Not *this* busy."

As Cheryl and I talked further, I began to hear more about the parts of her life that were painful. I had the strong impression that she was angry with her husband, a traveling sales agent who was often on the road and rarely home with her and the kids. "And when he is home," Cheryl went on, "he's usually either drinking or passed out cold. I'm not saying he has a problem—I know it's his way of relaxing—but sometimes I wonder. . . ." I wondered whether Cheryl was scared of what might happen if she really faced her suspicion that her husband *did* have a drinking problem. Perhaps her constant busyness was a way of never having the calm and quiet to ask herself how she really felt about her husband or to question the choices she was making.

Although Cheryl had done so many admirable things in her life, I had the impression that from her own point of view, it was never enough. She was quick enough to tell me about her accomplishments. But whenever I expressed my admiration, she made a face and told me about someone in her office, her neighborhood, or her profession who made Cheryl's achievements look minor by comparison. I had the feeling that despite her credentials, Cheryl didn't value herself much, and I wondered whether her parents had inadvertently given her the message that she'd never amount to anything, no matter what she did. Again, it seemed to me, Cheryl's busyness might be a way of not having to face these feelings.

Cheryl's busyness, her competitiveness, and perhaps also her low self-esteem were very much part of the culture of parenting she seemed to be in the midst of. I heard a great deal about how busy her children were, too, with homework and lessons and school clubs and sports. I asked Cheryl what would happen if the whole family took one day off just to spend time together, or if her children had after-school activities three days a week but were free the other two. Cheryl looked at me in astonishment.

"But then they'd be ostracized!" she told me. "They'd be completely different from all the other kids they go to school with. Everybody would be sure Woody and I were bad parents, or maybe they'd think we'd lost a lot of money, or . . . I wouldn't feel right, anyway, not giving them every advantage."

Cheryl left our appointment planning to start the adrenal-friendly diet and herbal supplements I suggested for her, and she promised to think about ways she could make some changes in her schedule. But I couldn't help feeling that there was an addictive quality to her busyness, a way that her minutely overscheduled life helped her keep disturbing thoughts and feelings at bay. There may even be a physically addictive aspect to that rush of stress hormones coursing through the body, so that without the constant buzz of being on high alert, life comes to seem a little boring. Many of us, myself included, have to contend with schedules that are too full, especially if we're balancing parenthood, other family responsibilities, and a full-time job. But where is the line between "I just have a lot to do" and "I'm afraid to give myself some downtime"?

I tried to help Cheryl think about her relationship to busyness, and now I'd like to do the same for you. Take the following quiz to find out whether being busy is making you happy—or simply wearing you out.

Are You Happy Being Busy?

Circle the number in front of any statement that seems true to you. Then look below to determine your score.

1. I look forward to most of my day and feel excited about what I do.

2. At the end of the day, I feel a strong sense of satisfaction and pride.

3. I often get anxious worrying about how much I have to do.

4. When I've finished a task, I find it difficult to pause and enjoy my accomplishment because I'm already on to the next task.

5. Most of the things I have to do during the day are boring or unpleasant.

6. I often wish I didn't have so much to do.

7. When I finish a project, I feel pleasure, excitement, or peace.

8. My idea of a great day off is just getting to sleep as much as I want to.

9. Starting a new project fills me with excitement.

10. Starting a new project fills me with dread.

11. Starting a new project leaves me cold—I don't really care.

12. When I go on vacation, I find myself frequently thinking about what I've left undone at home or work, and what I'll have to do when I get back.

13. I almost never take a vacation.

14. I live for the weekend.

15. I often end a weekend feeling more tired than when I began it.

16. When I picture a quiet day with nothing planned, I feel anxious.

17. When I picture a quiet day with nothing planned, I think about sleeping.

18. I often feel I could do better if I just worked a little harder.

19. Most of the time I feel proud of what I accomplish.

20. Sometimes I fantasize about just getting away from everything and going where nobody knows me and starting all over.

Give yourself 3 points for each of the following statements you circled: 1, 2, 7, 9, 19. Subtract 1 point for every other statement you chose.

- *10–15 points:* Congratulations. Even if you are busy, you basically enjoy your life and feel energized by it. Your attitude toward busyness will help you prevent adrenal dysfunction if you do not have it, and will help you overcome it if you do have it. To find further support and possible ways to improve, see Chapters 7 and 9 on lifestyle and the exploration of your emotions.

- *5–10 points:* You are ambivalent about the things you do. On the one hand, you feel pleasure and excitement in your activities; on the other hand, you often feel burdened, stressed, or overscheduled. Check out Chapters 7 and 9 for further suggestions that might help you feel less burdened and more excited about your life.

- *0–5 points:* You may feel frustrated with your busy life and it's hard for you to see a way out. Don't be discouraged. It can be challenging to reorganize your life and make your days more satisfying, but now that you've identified the problem, you're well on your way to creating a solution. Part II will offer you support for your mind, body, emotions, and spirit as you restore your energy and rediscover your joy in life.

- *Negative score:* You might find that so much of your life feels frustrating and overwhelming that it's hard for you to even think of making changes. I completely understand—but it doesn't have to be that way. Always know that you can change things. You will find a great deal of support in Part II for an adrenal-friendly eating plan to restore your energy, lifestyle changes that can support your health, and emotional work that can free you from some of the burdens you carry. Even a few baby steps can make a big difference, so don't give up.

Seeing Symptoms Progress

My patient Naomi was showing the first signs of adrenal dysfunction. A nurse at a local nursing-care facility in her early 30s, she was one of the most loving, caring people I'd ever met. Unlike many women, she had a good relationship with her body, and she seemed to have a strong sense of who she was.

But life threw several curves at Naomi, one after the other. First, her mother was diagnosed with lymphoma. Since Naomi's father had died several years earlier and since her siblings lived in other states, all of her mother's care fell on her: talking with the doctors, helping to make health-care decisions, visiting her mother in the hospital, offering moral support.

Then Naomi's 18-month-old daughter, Anya, was diagnosed with autism. Naomi and her husband began researching the disorder and trying to learn what they could do for Anya; but the combination of Naomi's stressful job, her mother's illness, and her daughter's diagnosis just proved to be too much. Naomi started getting one cold after another, gained ten pounds seemingly out of nowhere even though her diet hadn't changed, and for the first time in her life had trouble falling asleep at night. Normally a calm, cheerful person, Naomi found herself snapping at co-workers, yelling at her husband, and being brusque with her patients. She realized something was really wrong when she stopped just short of grabbing her daughter and squeezing her way too hard.

"I was just on the verge of snatching her out of her crib when I realized, 'Oh, my goodness, what is happening here?'" Naomi told me, her voice still shaky. "It was like I didn't even know what I was doing—like my body just took over. I realized that I wasn't willing to have my children be affected by this—but what can I do about it? What is *wrong* with me?"

I was so moved by what a big step Naomi was taking, confessing her fears to me and making changes that would affect how her children grew up. I congratulated Naomi on realizing that she needed help and reassured her that when we're facing the kinds of enormous stress that she was under, we often feel frayed and close to the edge. Sudden impulsive rage is characteristic of an amygdala reaction—an emotional reaction that bypasses the thoughtful, rational cerebral cortex and simply takes over our bodies before our minds have the chance to catch up. That Naomi had come so close to "losing it" showed how overly stressed she was.

Naomi's salivary cortisol tests and her other symptoms showed that she was experiencing only *mild* adrenal dysfunction at this point. She was at the "wired" stage when cortisol levels are almost constantly high with periodic crashes. I explained to Naomi that adrenal dysfunction is a progressive condition, and that if she didn't make some changes, she might find herself with symptoms of a *moderate* dysfunction and then, eventually, *severe* dysfunction.

Naomi looked at me fearfully. "Is that inevitable?" she asked. "How long do I have?"

There are never any easy answers to those questions. It's certainly possible that, depending on diet, lifestyle, genetics, and life events, a woman's symptoms can remain either *mild* or *moderate* indefinitely. Women who have the most adrenal-friendly diets and who nurture themselves emotionally are most likely to be able to stall the progress of the disorder.

Some women are actually able to overcome adrenal dysfunction while their symptoms are still *mild* or *moderate,* even if they don't completely follow the program I lay out in Part II or fully resolve their relationship to stress. If they, like Naomi, have been pushed into adrenal dysfunction by a number of real-life stressors and those stressors disappear—the trauma from the divorce fades, the ailing family member recovers—and if they have been eating in a healthy way and getting appropriate exercise and sleep, then it's possible that their condition will simply resolve itself. Suddenly they'll have more energy, find their excess weight easier to lose, and be able to return to a balanced state of health.

Other people, of course, will experience a rapid progression of adrenal symptoms, again for a number of reasons. I recently saw a patient who had extremely *severe* symptoms although she was barely 18 years old. She suffered from a significant gluten allergy that was compromising her thyroid function, and her adrenals were virtually exhausted. Even though she tested negative for Addison's disease, her adrenals were providing her system with such low levels of stress hormones that she could barely make it through the day. Fortunately, she was able to make several positive changes, including a gluten-free diet, which restored her to health within a few months.

So I couldn't really say what Naomi's prognosis would be. I could only tell her that she had gotten onto a path that led to a very poor outcome. How far or how fast she would travel down that path was hard to know.

Certainly Naomi was facing two major stressors—her mother's poor health and her daughter's autism diagnosis—along with the everyday stress of her demanding job. And, like almost everyone I know, she was also struggling with historical stress—in her case, a father who who was absent because he was working all the time and a mother who had enormously high expectations of her. Naomi always felt that she'd disappointed her mother by becoming "only" a nurse, and the burden of that disappointment added to her allostatic load.

When I looked at Naomi's life, I saw a woman who was breast-feeding the world. Whoever needed her—a family member, a friend, a colleague, a stranger—would get the absolute best that Naomi had to offer. As a result, Naomi had very little left to give herself. Naomi truly was a generous, loving person but her excessive caretaking was also a response to childhood experiences. Although Naomi's mother hadn't intended to give her this message, Naomi had come to understand that other people deserved care and she did not. So Naomi offered herself to everyone she could—and her adrenal dysfunction was at least partly the result.

The challenge Naomi faced was whether she wanted merely to stall the progress of her condition or whether she wanted to truly turn it around. An adrenal-friendly diet, the right herbal supplements, and appropriate exercise might be enough to keep her symptoms *mild*. Even so, her HPA axis would remain out of balance. Because there's so much cross talk between the HPA axis and the body's other systems, Naomi ran the risk of developing other problems, such as thyroid abnormalities, digestive difficulties, or problems with PMS or her menstrual periods.

Or Naomi could reverse her condition by working on all levels, including emotional reprogramming. Her challenge was to decide that she was worth it, and to give herself some of the same care she gave to everyone else.

"Look," I told Naomi, "you're dealing with so much right now. Please don't get down on yourself or think you have to change it all right away. Just being aware is a *huge* piece of the puzzle—and now you *are* aware. I am here to support you in whatever way I can, and I absolutely believe that you can find your own way—and your own pace—of turning things around."

It was not an option for Naomi to stop caring for either her mother or her daughter, so those major stressors would continue. But if she altered her relationship to historical stress—if she found a way to drop the burden of her mother's disappointment and live life on her own terms—everything else would get easier, including changing her diet, getting appropriate exercise, and finding *some* time for herself.

"I see what you mean," Naomi finally said. "Things won't get easy—they can't, as long as I'm dealing with Mom and Anya. But they can be *easier,* and that's the margin I need to turn things around." Once Naomi's attitude shifted, her internal messaging could shift as well, relieving the pressure on her HPA axis and beginning to ease her adrenal-related symptoms.

Burnout

Whether your symptoms are *mild, moderate,* or *severe,* if you've been living with chronic stress long enough, or if stress levels are intense enough, you may reach that emotional and physical state that is commonly known as burnout.

If you have *severe* symptoms, you're probably feeling burned out most of the time—plus you're exhausted. If your symptoms are *mild* or *moderate,* you may go in and out of feeling burned out, though you may also sometimes have the physical and emotional energy to accomplish a task or handle a situation gracefully. Far more often than you would like, however, you simply feel frayed. You may snap at people, lose your temper easily, and feel ready to dissolve into tears at the slightest challenge—a package you can't open, a permission slip you can't find, your preschooler unable to find her shoe.

I tell my patients—and myself!—that we know we're doing too much when we over-react. When something that's really minor seems major to us, that's a surefire sign that we've pushed ourselves too hard and we need a break, even if just a minute of breathing exercise is all we can manage. Start with where you are and do what you can.

Are you burned out? Take the following quiz and find out.

Are You Burned Out?

Choose the answer to each question that best describes the reaction you'd be most likely to have:

1. You're in the midst of getting ready for your daughter's birthday party and a dear friend who has done many favors for you calls. She's got an important doctor's appointment next week and wants your moral support, so she's asking you to go with her. You:

a.   Tell her that you'd be happy to go and assure her she doesn't have to worry about it anymore.

b.   Say "Yes" and feel resentful.

c.   Say, "I just can't think about this now, I'm sorry!" and hang up.

d.   Become hysterical and launch into a long list of all the things you have to get done between now and next week.

2. You're at work and your supervisor informs you that an already difficult deadline has been moved up. You:

  a. Explain calmly that the deadline was already too stringent and show why the new one can't possibly work.

  b. Just barely control your temper with your supervisor but then snap at your colleagues for the next few hours.

  c. Feel so low and discouraged that you begin to seriously consider quitting.

  d. Excuse yourself, run to the bathroom, and burst into tears.

3. All week you've been looking forward to a night out with your new romantic prospect, but at the last minute you get a call saying, "Sorry, Mom just had a minor cardiac episode. She's going to be fine, and my sister is here, but I feel I have to be here, too. I hate to cancel our date, but I don't think I have a choice." You:

  a. Say sincerely that you understand completely and offer your support.

  b. Express your frustration and disappointment, and then feel sorry afterward that you've done so.

  c. Hang up the phone and decide that the relationship is probably over now.

  d. Have a panic attack.

4. It's a major holiday and your relatives are all coming for dinner. It's potluck but you are making the turkey and many of the side dishes. Uncle Joe is supposed to bring the cranberry sauce but at the last minute he calls and says he can't make it— an old friend has come into town and Uncle Joe is going to spend time with him. You can only imagine what Aunt Martha and Cousin Jean will say if you serve turkey with no cranberry sauce, but you don't have time to run to the store and there's no one available to go. You:

  a. Shrug and say, "Either someone will run out for it after they get here, or we'll do without."

b.   Spend an hour cooking with one hand and frantically dialing the phone with the other, desperately trying to find someone to pick up the cranberry sauce on their way over.

   c.   Yell at Joe and tell him how inconsiderate he's being and how he's now ruined this holiday for the entire family.

   d.   Hang up and burst into tears.

5. You're trying to get the kids ready for the school bus when your son knocks over a glass and it breaks. You:

   a.   Say, "That's all right, honey, everyone makes mistakes. Let's get the broom and dustpan and clean it up."

   b.   Snap, "Why can't you be more careful!"

   c.   Yell, "I can't believe how you're always causing trouble!"

   d.   Launch into a five-minute tirade about how nobody in this house knows how to take care of anything and you just can't afford to keep replacing all the things that everyone keeps breaking.

- If most of your answers were (a), congratulations. You have a healthy perspective on life's daily challenges, and a good reserve of energy to deal with them.

- If many of your answers were (b), pay attention. You may be feeling a bit frayed.

- If many of your answers were (c), be careful. You're often reacting at a far higher pitch than the—admittedly challenging—situation warrants. You may sometimes—or often—feel burned out.

- If many of your answers were (d), you are operating under severe stress—and it shows. Even relatively small challenges are putting you over the edge. Take steps to either reduce the stress in your life, change your relationship to stress, or, ideally, both.

Still not sure whether you're burned out? Take a look at the following checklist. How many of these descriptions sound like you? If you find yourself nodding in recognition, you may well be taking on too much.

- ☐ While you're driving, someone pulls out in front of you and, five miles later, you're still simmering with annoyance, thinking of all the ways you'd like to tell the guy off.

- ☐ Your child spills grape juice on your favorite blouse and you're not sure the cleaners will be able to get the stain out. You feel as though your day has been ruined.

- ☐ When people ask you how you are, you find yourself saying, "Fried," "Too busy," "Tired," or simply "Numb."

- ☐ At least one friend or family member has accused you of "always snapping at me" or of being impatient.

- ☐ You find yourself frequently losing your temper with clerks, waitstaff, and customer-service representatives on the phone.

- ☐ When you stand in a slow-moving line, you find yourself monitoring the behavior of the people in front of you and steaming about why they don't move more quickly.

Turning It All Around

As we have seen, adrenal dysfunction is a progressive condition. The good news, though, is that you can absolutely turn the process around. You only need to adopt an adrenal-friendly diet, a lifestyle that reduces the stress in your life, and a commitment to reworking your approach to historical and present-day stress. You can find the support for all those solutions in Part II—so let's get started.

ADRENAL-FRIENDLY ACTIVITIES: WAYS TO BEGIN TO HEAL

- *Reserve a family TV or movie night.* Spend some quality time with your children doing something they like—and can talk to you about afterward. Take turns picking a movie that the whole family will enjoy, or choose a TV show that you can watch with one or more of your children. The only rule is "No electronic communication when the TV is on," so your kids can't text or make cell-phone calls as if you weren't there. Watching something they enjoy also gives you a chance to learn more about them, and maybe even hear them express an opinion or two during or after the show. Make it a regular thing, so your kids know they can count on a time when they'll have your undivided attention, should they need it—or when they can just enjoy hanging out with you.

- *Move more.* Go for a walk or a bike ride in a neighborhood or park that you enjoy. Even five or ten minutes spent moving and enjoying your surroundings can make a huge difference to your morale.

- *Spend time with friends.* Study after study has shown that people in loving, supportive social networks do far better healthwise than people who are isolated. Even in the midst of your crazy schedule, make time to have lunch with a good friend.

- *Listen to music.* Music can be a terrific way to cue our bodies to calm down. Find some tracks you like and give yourself at least five minutes to listen to a beloved song or a piece of instrumental music.

PART II

Your Solution to Adrenal Dysfunction: 30 Days to Feel Like Yourself Again

YOUR SOLUTION TO ADRENAL DYSFUNCTION: YOUR 30-DAY PLAN

- Follow an adrenal-friendly diet.

- Follow the individualized dietary supplement recommendations for your adrenal type.

- Get moderate, regular amounts of gentle exercise.

- Engage in a de-stress practice: yoga, meditation, or conscious relaxation.

- Be good to yourself.

- Identify the emotional issues—often stemming from childhood—that create additional stress and find a way to work through them.

Now that you understand more about adrenal dysfunction, I hope you're eager to begin your own mind-body solution, a 30-day plan that will have you feeling significantly better in just weeks. When you're feeling low in body and spirit, it can be hard to believe that you'll ever feel like yourself again. So before we look at the specifics, I want to tell you what I tell my patients: *Change is possible.* It truly is. I know that if you've been struggling with adrenal dysfunction for months or perhaps years, you may be feeling discouraged. You may have tried weight-loss plans that didn't work, exercise regimens that just wore you out, and anti-stress routines that didn't actually relieve your stress.

But there were good reasons why those previous approaches didn't work—and there are good reasons why this one can. Over the past two decades, I've treated thousands of patients with adrenal dysfunction, and I've seen it time and again: within a month, things start to improve. Within two months, many symptoms disappear. And within three months or more, virtually all of my patients are well on their way to fully restoring adrenal balance, regearing their metabolism, and regaining their natural energy. That can be your story, too.

DIET AND
SUPPLEMENTS

Annette had struggled with weight all her life, and when she came to me at age 45, she was extremely frustrated. "Diets just don't work for me," she said, staring at me with a look that dared me to disagree. "I've tried every one—Atkins, South Beach, the Zone, and a bunch of others—and the only one that has come close is Weight Watchers. And even then, I have to worry about every bite of every meal, and if I make one little slip, I gain it all back. I know it's not healthy for me to carry this extra 15 pounds, and I hate the way it makes me feel. But honestly, I've given up hope."

As Annette and I talked, I began to suspect that her adrenals were at the root of the problem. After questioning her more extensively and ordering the usual tests, I was able to confirm my initial diagnosis: Annette was suffering from what was virtually a textbook case of adrenal dysfunction. She ate irregularly and often missed meals. She usually skipped breakfast and rushed through lunch. Her biggest meal of the day was dinner, which she tended to have an hour or two before bedtime. Equally important, her life was one long, frantic round of activities. Her job, her kids, her husband, and her volunteer work left her with virtually no time for herself.

Together, Annette and I worked out how she could alter her habits to follow an adrenal-friendly diet. My suggestions included:

- Regular mealtimes and snack times, eating approximately every three hours, with the first meal taken within an hour of rising.

- The biggest meal taken early in the day, with dinner being the lightest meal.

- No food within three hours of bedtime.

- No processed sugar, "white foods" (processed flour, breads, or pasta), caffeine, or alcohol.

- A gluten-free diet that contained no wheat, rye, barley, or oats (except certified gluten-free oats, such as Bob's Red Mill).

- Herbal supplements tailored to Annette's particular form of adrenal dysfunction.

- Gentle exercise three times a week.

- A minimum of seven hours of sleep each night.

- At least 15 minutes each day devoted entirely to herself.

Initially Annette understood the food-and-exercise portion of the plan. She wasn't so sure about the sleep and personal-time requirements. I explained to her that every aspect of the plan was designed to restore and rebalance her adrenals so that they could help her body reach the healthiest possible weight. I believe that it's easier to follow an eating plan if you know why you're following it. So let's look at each aspect of the adrenal-friendly eating plan and see how it's going to help rebalance your system and heal your adrenals.

Myths and Facts about Your Weight

It never ceases to amaze me how many myths we're bombarded with concerning diet, exercise, and weight. Following are some common myths that I hear frequently from my patients. Have you heard them, too? Have you begun to realize that they're false?

Myth: Cutting fat and calories is all you need to do to lose weight.

Fact: A low-fat, low-calorie diet is not good for most women. The quality of the food you eat is the key factor in a healthy diet. Food is information. Your adrenal imbalance is also a nutritional imbalance. Your body is craving certain types of nutrients and, without them, your adrenals can't function properly. And if your adrenals aren't functioning properly, you'll find it very difficult to lose weight. Since we've gone low-fat/no-fat, obesity rates have actually increased. So make sure you get the good-quality fats that you need, or you may actually gain weight.

Myth: Vigorous exercise is beneficial to any weight-loss program.

Fact: If you're suffering from adrenal imbalance, too much exertion will actually have the opposite effect, raising your stress levels and driving your body to produce more cortisol, which will contribute to fatigue as well as interfere with your weight loss. Depending on your adrenals, moderate or gentle exercise may be better for you, at least for a while.

Myth: It doesn't matter what kind of food you eat, as long as it's low-fat or low-calorie.

Fact: Different food has different impacts on different body types. The quality of the food is crucial, since food speaks to your genes. If you don't address the hormonal imbalances that are driving your weight gain, just reducing caloric intake won't help. Your body will continue to produce cortisol, a hormone that drives your body to hold on to fat, as well as create other metabolic imbalances.

Myth: After menopause, it's pretty much inevitable that you gain five pounds each year.

Fact: Although many women do gain weight after menopause, that is by no means inevitable. Postmenopausal weight gain—like premenopausal weight gain—is often the result of adrenal imbalances that have never been attended to and have simply gotten worse with age. When the adrenals are balanced, the weight returns to a healthy level.

Myth: If you're overweight when you go into menopause, you need an hour a day of exercise just to maintain your current weight.

Fact: If you're overweight, you may need more exercise—but you don't need to drive yourself nearly that hard. In fact, doing so may make your body think, "Emergency!" and hold on to your body fat even harder. If you've tried a healthy diet and moderate exercise and still failed to lose weight, your body is probably out of balance in some way. You may be struggling with hormonal issues, insulin resistance, thyroid abnormalities, adrenal dysfunction, or some combination of all of these. Find the problem and solve it. Don't push yourself to higher levels of exertion.

Myth: You can't rehabilitate your metabolism. Once it's slow, it's slow.
Fact: Your metabolism is extremely responsive to diet, exercise, and adrenal function. Getting your adrenals into tip-top condition can work wonders with resetting your metabolism and then keeping it healthy.

Timing Is Everything

Timing your meals and snacks may well be the most important aspect of the adrenal-friendly eating plan:

- Plan for regular mealtimes and snack times, eating approximately every three hours, with the first meal taken within an hour of rising.

- Eat your biggest meal early in the day, with dinner being the lightest meal.

- Stop eating three hours before bedtime.

There are two reasons for this plan. First, getting too hungry means you've let your blood-sugar levels drop—and low blood sugar stresses your body and can tax your adrenals. In fact, your body and your brain are in constant need of energy in the form of blood sugar, even as you sleep. Cortisol—one of the stress hormones released by your adrenals—makes sure your blood sugar stays high enough to feed your body's muscles and organs. This is especially important at night, so that you don't become depleted while you sleep. So when you've gone for a while without eating—as you must when you're sleeping!—cortisol signals your liver to release *stored* sugar, called *glycogen*.

The adrenals are strong enough to do this during the hours that you're sleeping—but they're not really designed to keep doing it all day long, too. Long periods without food make the adrenals work harder—they have to release more cortisol to signal your liver to release glycogen. As we've seen, if you're living a stressful life, your adrenals are working pretty hard already, releasing cortisol in response to deadlines; your children's crises; and perhaps also your own anxieties, fears, and frustrations. While we're working on calming your whole system down, let's not make your adrenals work any harder than they have to! Keep your body well supplied with blood sugar by eating every three hours, and give your adrenals a rest.

The other key reason for timing your meals has to do with your cortisol cycle. As we've seen in previous chapters, cortisol has a natural cycle that works with your circadian rhythm. Normally, cortisol begins to rise around 6:00 A.M., peaks at 8 A.M., and then gradually declines throughout the day, apart from small rises in response to exercise, meals, or snacks. At night, healthy cortisol levels are usually low, in preparation for nighttime rest. It's ideal to work with this natural cycle to avoid dramatic ups and downs. The best way to do this is to get most of your food in earlier in the day and to eat an early dinner, by 6 P.M.

Most of my patients have trouble doing this, especially if they work outside the home. And you might recall that I suggested delaying your own evening meal a bit further if you have young children, so that you can sit with them while they eat but then consume your own dinner in a more restful atmosphere. That's all fine—just try to make your evening meal the lightest one of the day, to prevent a surge of cortisol from ramping up your nighttime metabolic rate and disrupting your ability to fall or stay asleep. And if even this is too difficult, don't worry—just do your best.

Many of my patients tell me they overeat in the evening to soothe themselves, especially those who fit the Workhorse profile we saw in Chapter 3. If they've been living with high levels of stress all day, their cortisol is quite high—and that can either stimulate or decrease their appetites. This can lead to the vicious cycle that we saw before: if stress stimulates the appetite, then nighttime eating disturbs sleep, and the Workhorse becomes exhausted—and her next day is all the more stressful. If she uses caffeine to keep herself going through that exhausted day, she's compounding the problem even further, as the caffeine in her system will also help keep her awake. One way to "get off the merry-go-round" is to shift eating patterns, with the heaviest meal in the morning, the lightest one at night, and either no caffeine or very restricted caffeine during the day. (We'll learn more about caffeine in a moment.)

Keep in mind that cortisol will also rise a bit with exercise. Lighter activities, such as a walk after dinner or a bit of gentle stretching before bedtime, will not subvert this natural tapering-off process. But to work in concert with your body's natural cortisol cycle, more intense exercise is often best planned for the morning, before you eat. However, listen to your body's symphony: Some of my patients prefer to exercise at the end of the day, sometime between 4 P.M. and 7 P.M., to release the day's stress. I personally prefer to exercise in the morning, but again, there's no one right way. You should decide when exercise feels best to you and plan to do it then. The ideal is to not push and to check in with yourself. If you feel fabulous after a workout, then you've found the ideal time. If you feel exhausted, you need to either find another time or perhaps wait until your adrenals are in better shape.

Here, then, is the ideal eating schedule to support your body's natural cortisol cycle:

- If possible, eat breakfast by 7 A.M. or within an hour of getting up (a half hour after waking is even better), to restore blood-sugar levels after using glycogen stores at night.

- Aim for a nutritious snack around 10 A.M. to keep your blood sugar stable.

- Try to eat lunch between noon and 1 P.M. Your morning meal and snack can be used up quickly.

- Eat a nutritious snack between 2 P.M. and 3 P.M. to get you through the natural dip in cortisol around 3 P.M. or 4 P.M.

- Make an effort to eat dinner by 6 P.M. and make this your lightest meal of the day.

Supporting your body's natural rhythms by timing meals every three hours and preventing dramatic dips in blood sugar will help ensure that your body isn't flooded with excess cortisol. At the same time, it will contribute to rebalancing your adrenals and help them to heal. You'll notice almost immediately that eating this way gives you more sustained energy throughout the day—and life becomes much more enjoyable when we have all the energy we need.

But I'm Not Hungry in the Morning

As your mother probably told you, breakfast is important. But maybe you don't feel hungry in the morning.

There are two possible reasons for that morning lack of appetite, and either or both might apply to you. The first has to do with the cascade of hormones set off by the HPATGG axis. Remember that the hypothalamus signals the pituitary to signal the adrenal glands to send out more stress hormones as it gets light outside, so that our body will begin to rev up and awaken. The hypothalmus's signal is sent via a biochemical called corticotropin-releasing hormone (CRH), which tends to dull your appetite.

Even if you don't feel hungry, I urge you to have a nutritious breakfast within an hour of rising, preferably with protein. Your metabolism will kick back into gear more quickly, your cortisol levels will stay even, and your adrenals will heal far more quickly. More energy and faster weight loss will also result.

Calm Your System Down

I suggest cutting out sugar, "white foods" (processed flour, breads, or pasta), caffeine, or alcohol, which tend to play havoc with your blood-sugar levels. When you consume refined sweets or starchy foods, your blood sugar rises quickly and for a little while, you feel a surge of energy. But because these foods are metabolized so quickly, that "sugar high" is soon followed by a crash. Your liver, pancreas, and adrenals are working overtime again, trying to even out your blood sugar, supplying extra cortisol to get those blood-sugar levels back up, and contributing to your stress levels. Eating foods that are metabolized more slowly—proteins, whole grains, and some vegetables—helps keep your blood sugar on an even keel, giving your adrenals some much-needed rest. You also want to eat more low-glycemic foods—foods that are not converted as quickly to sugar—since that, too, will keep your blood sugar stable and help your adrenals to heal. (For a list of low- and high-glycemic foods, see Appendix C.)

Too many sweet or starchy foods can also create *insulin resistance,* a prediabetic condition that makes it much harder to lose weight. Insulin is a key hormone produced by the pancreas that allows glucose to travel from the bloodstream into the cells, where it helps cells function. As we just saw, sweet and starchy foods raise your blood-sugar level quickly. In response, your insulin level surges to remove that sugar from your blood and get it into your cells. If this happens only occasionally, there's no problem. But if your blood sugar—and therefore your insulin—spikes too often, your cells respond by decreasing the reactivity and number of insulin receptors on their surfaces, causing the insulin to be "resistant" to doing its job. Eventually, this prevents glucose from getting into your cells. You end up with chronically high blood sugar, even as your cells are deprived of the energy they need to function.

This is why many women with insulin resistance experience carb cravings, fatigue, and weight gain. Their cells are literally starving for energy, even when plenty of glucose is available in the blood. The long-term danger is that all those insulin surges deplete your body's capacity to generate insulin, potentially setting you up for type 2 diabetes.

The solution is to eat foods that allow for a slower, gentler rise in insulin levels because they take more time to digest—in other words, whole fresh foods that are rich in protein, complex carbohydrates, and nutrients. Exercise can also help reverse or prevent insulin resistance because it increases the insulin receptors on your cells. (You'll find suggestions for your exercise plan in Chapter 7.)

Like sugar, caffeine—found in coffee, caffeinated tea, chocolate, soda, energy drinks (such as Red Bull), and ma huang or ephedra (used in weight-loss supplements)—also gives you a quick burst of energy. But it too can overstimulate the adrenals, further exhausting these overworked glands and making you feel even more tired when the caffeine wears off. Caffeine may also keep you up at night, unless you restrict your caffeine intake to mornings or early afternoons. The half-life of caffeine in the body ranges from three and a half to six hours.

Even after you fall asleep, caffeine can make your sleep less restful. Instead of allowing your blood vessels to dilate, which allows more oxygen into the brain as you sleep, caffeine constricts your blood vessels, keeping you from getting all the oxygen you need. Incidentally, too much coffee or soda may be part of why you wake up feeling tired— and then reach for another coffee or soda.

Of course, caffeine can also make you feel wonderful! That's because it triggers an upswing in a biochemical called dopamine, which activates the pleasure center in the brain. Would it surprise you to know that's just what cocaine, amphetamines, and other psychoactive drugs do? And some research even shows that small amounts of caffeine can be beneficial.

The problem is that caffeine also triggers an upswing in cortisol and other stress hormones—and we've seen how much damage that can do, especially when you have "tired and wired" adrenals. As with other types of chronic stress, the problem is twofold. First, because of all the cross talk between the HPA axis and the body's other systems, the excess stress hormones cause all sorts of physical problems, including potential problems for your thyroid, gut, and sex hormones. They also interfere with your sleep, make you feel anxious and "wired," and leave you feeling tired when they wear off. Furthermore, after too many years of overstimulation, your adrenal reserves become exhausted. No longer "tired and wired," you end up just plain tired.

As I explained in *The Core Balance Diet,* caffeine tolerance varies from woman to woman, depending on how efficiently her liver "detoxifies" the caffeine and removes it from her system. Because caffeine is a habit-forming drug, you usually need more and more of it to produce the same effects, so it's difficult for many people to keep their caffeine intake at a steady level, especially if other aspects of their life, diet, or physical condition are exhausting them.

If you find yourself craving caffeine—or sugar, for that matter—it may be that your cortisol is low, but it also simply may be that your body needs to rest. I encourage you to honor your body's request and take a break, instead of winding it up another notch. Take a quiet moment and treat yourself to some deep breathing or a ten-minute walk.

If you are an efficient detoxifier, caffeine itself may not be a problem. But if you're struggling with adrenal dysfunction, it can certainly complicate your healing process, and it may very well be part of the cycle that's making you ever more wired or tired. My suggestion would be to cut out caffeine entirely for your 30-day adrenal-friendly diet and see how your body responds, promising yourself that you can resume caffeine in moderation if you still want to at the month's end. You may discover that you actually don't want to. At the very least, you'll become more sensitive to the effects of caffeine upon your body and can then make better choices about when and how much you want to consume. And if drinking a cup of coffee is a relaxing part of your routine that you don't want to give up, drink it in the morning with something nutritious to eat, including some healthy protein, and add milk or cream to dull the negative effects of the caffeine.

Basically, the same is true for tea. Tea can be very beneficial, especially green tea, but it can also push your system past the healthy point. Listen to your body and make the choices that are right for you.

Likewise, even decaf diet soda can be problematic because it usually contains Splenda, which in the processing becomes something similar to chlorinated sugar. I strongly suggest avoiding these types of drinks, or at least limiting them as much as possible.

I advise against alcohol, too. Because it's a depressant, it usually includes a fair amount of sugar and relaxes your inhibitions, often making it difficult to stay on a healthy eating plan. A glass or two of wine won't kill you once in a while, but I strongly counsel against daily drinking, especially while you're trying to help your adrenals to heal. Again, new research shows that six ounces of red wine each day can be good for you—but not when your adrenals need to recover.

Overcoming Addictions:
Caffeine, Sugar, and Compulsive Behaviors

Many of us struggle with difficulty in letting go of our reliance on caffeine, our attraction to sugar, or our sometimes compulsive behaviors. While we tend to think of these struggles as an issue of willpower, there is often a biochemical basis. As a result, the correct supplements can frequently help us balance our systems and go a long way toward helping us to overcome our addictions.

Caffeine Dependence

To detox from caffeine, consider giving up your coffee or caffeinated sodas a little at a time rather than quitting cold turkey. If you're a coffee drinker, start the day with your regular cup of coffee, but for your second cup, try half-caf, half-decaf. Or, if you drink coffee and soda all day long, try a half-caf, half-decaf formula throughout the day.

Another option is to restrict your caffeine intake to mornings only, so that the stimulation you get mirrors your cortisol cycle. Some people do an "on-again, off-again" rhythm, with a few caffeine-free days each month to make sure their bodies don't become too dependent. You can also try drinking a big glass of pure water or a cup of herbal tea as soon as you wake up. Eat your breakfast as soon as possible, making sure to include adequate protein, and only then turn to your usual caffeinated drink, which you may not even want once your hunger and thirst are quenched.

Often, people have withdrawal symptoms as they give up caffeine, including headaches, fatigue, sluggishness, drowsiness, difficulty focusing, irritability, depression, anxiety, and a reduced sense of well-being. The symptom I see most often is headaches, and if you get these as you cut back on caffeine, that's a sign that you almost certainly are addicted to it. Headaches and any other symptoms usually peak within two to four days and should be gone within a single caffeine-free week. Support your body with extra vitamin C, regular breaks, a refreshing walk, and plenty of sleep, with regular sleep times and wake times. You can also try white willow bark tablets, which contain a natural type of pain-relieving salicylate. (Like aspirin, however, salicylates are derived from willow and should be avoided for two weeks before and after any surgery because of their blood-thinning effect.) Generally, you can support your liver—the organ that removes the caffeine from your system—with the following supplements:

- Amino acids (which may also help balance energy levels)

- B vitamins

- Vitamin C

- Calcium

- Magnesium

- Milk thistle

- N-acetyl cysteine

- Potassium

- Trace minerals

- Zinc

Sugar Cravings and Addictive Behaviors

Although our cravings and addictive behaviors feel real to us, they often are based on an imbalance of brain chemicals known as *neurotransmitters* that help us process emotions and information. Restoring the proper biochemical balance to our brains often makes a world of difference in the way we think and feel. Look for a supplement that contains such biochemicals as 5-HTP, N-acetylcysteine, L-DOPA, and L-phenylalanine, vitamin C, vitamin B_{12}, and B_6. Many companies make compounds that are very helpful in overcoming sugar cravings and addictive behaviors of all types. (See Resources for more information.)

DRINK YOUR WAY TO ADRENAL HEALTH

Your beverage choices can either support your adrenals or serve to exhaust them further. Here's a quick look at adrenal beverage dos and don'ts:

Adrenal Draining Beverages	Adrenal Restoring Beverages
Caffeinated drinks	Ginseng [Panax sp.] (in the morning)
Alcohol	Eleuthero/Siberian ginseng [*Eleutherococcus senticosus*] (in the morning)
Sugared sodas	Herbal teas such as chamomile, passionflower, valerian
Energy drinks	Licorice tea (in the morning), unless you, like the Racehorse, are wired
Gatorade	Vegetable juice (with salt), such as V8 or generic store brands
	Mineral water, such as S.Pellegrino or Perrier

Get Rid of the Gluten

Gluten is a complement of proteins found in grains, including wheat, rye, and barley. Thanks to cross-contamination in manufacturing, it is also found in most types of oats. Gluten is an ingredient in soy sauces, is frequently used as a food additive, and can be found in many other places that you might never suspect, such as in cosmetics containing wheat germ or wheat oil protein. You might discover that you have no problem with gluten, but I've found in my practice that many women with adrenal dysfunction are indeed sensitive to gluten, as are women with thyroid abnormalities. As we have seen, because of the cross talk along the HPATGG axis, thyroid problems and adrenal dysfunction often go hand in hand.

For these reasons, a gluten-free diet is one of the first things I suggest to patients with symptoms of adrenal dysfunction. Many of them, including Annette, the 45-year-old frustrated dieter, report that they feel much better when they get the gluten out of their diets.

If you're not sure about whether gluten is a problem for you, I suggest you cut it out entirely during your 30-day adrenal-friendly eating plan. Then, if you'd like to start eating whole grains that might contain glutens (because I'd like you to stay away from white and refined flours of all types), slowly introduce a gluten-containing food back into your diet. Pay attention—do you notice feeling more tired, foggy, forgetful, or otherwise "off"? If so, it might very well be the gluten, and you might consider keeping it out of your diet permanently.

A naturopath or functional-medicine specialist may be able to help you determine whether you have gluten sensitivity. Meanwhile, in the Resources section I offer some suggestions for where to order gluten-free products.

I know I'm asking you to make a lot of changes, so if this one feels overwhelming, just skip it for now. Do what's possible and let the rest go. My goal is to help you feel healthy and relaxed, not to make things more stressful for you.

Helpful Herbs

Most herbal supplements won't help directly with weight loss, but they will help to restore your adrenal reserves, giving you some more physical, mental, and emotional energy to recover your balance and move forward in your life. Some practitioners I know refuse to prescribe herbal supplements because they are concerned that as soon as a patient feels better, she'll run right out and overschedule her life again, avoiding the kinds of changes that will really heal her adrenals in the long run.

It's true that if you are really looking to feel better for the long term—to achieve your ideal weight and stay there, to approach your life with joy and vigor, to feel like yourself again—you're probably going to have to address the issues that threw you out of balance in the first place. If you're suffering from a physical problem, such as chronic pain, frequent infections, an environmental sensitivity, or an autoimmune disease, you'll want to address that condition as best you can, so that it doesn't continue to stress your adrenals. If you're suffering from real-life or historical stress, you'll need to change your situation and your relationship to stress so that you're making more time for yourself, being kinder to yourself, and making sure you get the emotional and spiritual support you need.

It's easier to accomplish all of those tasks if you've got a bit more energy, so I suggest adding herbal supplements and nutrients to your adrenal-friendly eating plan. *Always check with your doctor before taking any supplements, especially if you are on any other type of medication.* You might also want to work with a naturopath or functional-medicine practitioner to develop a course of herbal supplements tailored specifically to your needs. If your current doctor approves, here are some suggestions to get you started. Note that these recommendations are geared to the Racehorse, Workhorse, and Flatliner, which we identified in Chapter 3.

All Types:

These are basic nutrients to supplement a healthy diet:

- Omega-3 essential fatty acids, in the form of fish oil or krill oil

- A good multivitamin

- Calcium and magnesium supplements

If you buy fish oil, make sure you get the kind that is labeled "lead- and mercury-free." Know the company, and also make sure the fish oil is "pharmaceutical grade."

If you buy a multivitamin, try to approximate the following ingredients and doses for a daily total:

- Vitamin A, 10,000.00 IU

- Vitamin C, 1,200 mg

- Vitamin D, 400 IU

- Vitamin E, 200 IU

- Thiamin, 30 mg

- Riboflavin, 34 mg

- Niacin, 420 mg

- Vitamin B_6, 40 mg

- Folate, 800 mcg

- Vitamin B_{12}, 200 mcg

- Biotin, 200 mcg

- Pantothenic acid, 200 mg

- Calcium, 500 mg

- Iodine, 150 mcg

- Magnesium, 250 mg

- Zinc, 20 mg

- Selenium, 200 mcg

- Copper, 2 mg

- Manganese, 1 mg

- Chromium, 200 mcg

- Molybdenum, 100 mcg

- Potassium, 99 mg

- Betaine HCl, 175 mg

- Choline, 125 mg

- Inositol, 120 mg

- Citrus bioflavonoid complex, 100 mg

- Para-aminobenzoic acid (PABA), 50 mg

- Quercetin, 25 mg

- Mixed carotenoids (including beta-carotene, alpha-carotene, cryptoxanthin, zeaxanthin, and lutein), 5.85 mg

- Gamma-tocopherol, 67 mg

If you buy a calcium-magnesium supplement, try to approximate the following ingredients and doses:

- Calcium, 600 mg

- Magnesium, 300 mg

- Phosphorus, 378 mg

- Vitamin D, 600 IU

Don't take more than 1,500 mg of calcium daily—generally magnesium is half the amount of calcium. But some individuals need equal amounts of calcium and magnesium daily.

Make sure you also check your vitamin D status with your practitioner. If it's low, be sure to supplement with vitamin D as well, since your body needs D to help its calcium absorption as well as for many other health reasons.

If you have not yet entered menopause, look for a multivitamin that also includes iron (10 mg). If you're in menopause, you won't need the extra iron.

For the Racehorse:

To help balance your system, try these herbal supplements:

- Astragalus, one 400-mg to 470-mg capsule up to three times a day, or take an adaptogenic complex that includes some of the following herbs: rhodiola, cordyceps, and ashwagandha

- Royal maca, two to six 500-mg tablets each day

- Vitamin C, 500 mg (if you're not already taking vitamin C supplements)

To quiet your system and help you sleep, or to calm an agitated and pounding heart:

- A phosphorylated serine combination consisting of such ingredients as calcium (105 mg), magnesium (105 mg), phosphorus (355 mg), and l-serine (105 mg)

For the Workhorse:

To boost your energy, try these herbal supplements:

- Astragalus, one 400-mg to 470-mg capsule up to three times a day, or take an adaptogenic complex that includes some of the following herbs: rhodiola, cordyceps, and ashwagandha

- Siberian ginseng (unless you have high blood pressure), one 370-mg to 420-mg capsule, one to three times each day

To improve mood and immune function, build muscle, burn fat, and help with weight loss:

- DHEA, which can be found at health-food stores. You can also have it compounded to take under the supervision of a functional-medicine practitioner. I use DHEA drops, 1 mg per drop. I have my patients start with one drop, twice a day, and if they seem to need more, I increase the dosage each week by one drop in the morning and one drop in the evening, until they've reached five drops twice a day.

To help you sleep:

- A phosphorylated serine combination consisting of such ingredients as calcium (105 mg), magnesium (105 mg), phosphorus (355 mg), and l-serine (105 mg)

For the Flatliner:

To boost your energy, try these herbal supplements:

- Astragalus, one 400-mg to 470-mg capsule up to three times a day, or take an adaptogenic complex that includes some of the following herbs: rhodiola, cordyceps, and ashwagandha

- Siberian ginseng (unless you have high blood pressure), one 370-mg to 420-mg capsule, one to three times each day after meals

- Licorice root tea or extracts up to three times daily (unless you have high blood pressure)

To improve mood and immune function, build muscle, burn fat, and help with weight loss:

- DHEA, which can be found at health-food stores. You can also have it compounded to take under the supervision of a functional-medicine practitioner. I use DHEA drops, 1 mg per drop. I have my patients start with two drops, twice a day, and if they seem to need more, I increase their dosage one drop at a time until they've reached five drops twice a day.

If you feel that you've simply "hit the wall," and even these supplements aren't helping you boost your energy to a sufficient level, you might want to add to your daily intake a product such as Isocort, a freeze-dried adrenal cortex extract containing herbs and medium-chain triglycerides. I recommend that my patients take two tablets before breakfast, and two tablets before lunch. However, I strongly recommend taking this substance *only under the guidance of a functional-medical practitioner or naturopath. Please don't self-medicate with this product.*

THE HERBAL PHARMACY: DIGESTIVE ISSUES

Because of all the cross talk along the HPATGG axis, people with adrenal dysfunction often suffer from gastrointestinal problems. Here are some herbal supplements that might help. *Again, check with your doctor before taking any of the following supplements, and/or work with a naturopath or functional-medicine specialist to tailor solutions for your own needs.*

For bloating immediately after a meal:

- Try Swedish bitters

OR

- Betaine HCl (hydrochloric acid), beginning with one tablet after a meal and continuing to add tablets up to a total of three unless you feel a burning sensation, in which case you should cut back by one tablet (take for one or two months only). Do not take if you are taking a proton inhibitor or have a history of ulcers. Consult with your health-care practitioner.

For gas or bloating one or two hours after a meal:

- Try a compound that includes protease I (20,000 PC), protease II (200,000 USP), protease III (40,000 HUT), amylase (20,000 DU), lipase (2,000 LU), cellulase (2,000 CU), peptidase (600 units), maltase (600 DP), lactase (400 LAC U), invertase (400 SUMNER), and amla fruit (40 mg). Many companies make products with these ingredients. (For more information, see Resources.)

For indigestion:

- Try betaine HCl (hydrochloric acid). Begin with one tablet after a meal and continue to add tablets up to a total of three unless you feel a burning sensation, in which case you should cut back by one tablet. Try this regime for one to two months. If burning begins in your digestive tract, cut back the dose or stop altogether. Avoid this product if you have a history of ulcers or are on a proton pump inhibitor.

For constipation:

- Magnesium, 200 to 600 mg: Experiment with the dose but decrease if you develop diarrhea. Magnesium is also helpful for muscle spasms in the legs and feet.

For general digestive support:

- L-glutamine, 1,000 mg, one to three tablets three times a day to help heal digestive complaints. (Avoid if you have a bipolar disorder.)

- A probiotic, 10 billion CFU to 25 billion CFU several times a day, before meals, for a total of 20 billion CFU to 75 billion CFU per day. The more digestive complaints you have, the more probiotic you should take.

Even if you don't need the other supplements, I strongly urge you to take daily doses of a probiotic. By age two, we have established for life our intestinal flora—the bacteria we need to help digest our food and absorb nutrients. If our early years were stressed or undernourished, we probably need to supplement later in life. Since two-thirds of our serotonin—our natural "feel-good" antidepressant—is produced in the gut, any issue with digestion can lead to depression and also further stress our adrenals.

Sleep Your Way to a Healthy Weight

Get a minimum of seven hours of sleep each night. The connection between lack of sleep and weight retention is clear: insufficient sleep stresses your body; chronic loss of sleep equals chronic stress; and chronic stress means chronically high levels of cortisol, which encourages your body to hold on to every extra ounce of fat. If you regularly go without at least seven hours of good, restful sleep, you are going to find it nearly impossible to lose weight or even to maintain a healthy weight. I'll talk more about how to improve your sleep in Chapter 7, but meanwhile, commit to getting seven hours of sleep every night.

By the way, if you're regularly going without sleep, you can't really make up for it on the weekends. Every night without sleep is still a significant stressor, cuing your HPATGG axis to begin the biochemical cascade that floods your body with stress hormones. That's why people on shift work are so vulnerable to adrenal dysfunction; they find it very difficult to get good sleep when they're working an overnight or evening shift. An occasional off night is no big deal, but regularly missed sleep will stress your body no matter what you do on Saturday or Sunday.

Give Yourself a Break

Devote at least 15 minutes each day to yourself. I consider this an essential part of an adrenal-friendly eating plan for two reasons. First, as we've seen, chronic stress contributes significantly to weight retention. If we're going to lose the weight that's gained from adrenal dysfunction, we need to address the sources of chronic stress in our lives. And if even the idea of taking 15 minutes for yourself each day fills you with anxiety or despair, then you are almost certainly living a life that is filled with chronic stress.

I know it's hard to find even a few minutes a day to focus on yourself, especially if you have a demanding job, a family—or, most especially, both. I don't think I did a particularly good job of balancing my needs with my family's needs and my patients' needs as my own children were growing up (they're young adults now), and I see how hard this balancing act is for almost all of my patients. But I believe that if we *don't* find ways to care for ourselves in the midst of our challenging lives, we're going to have an extremely hard time restoring our health, reaching an appropriate weight, and enjoying the vigor and energy to which we are entitled.

Second, it's when we feel worst about ourselves and our lives that many of us turn to food for comfort. These negative messages almost always come from our history— from parents who, perhaps without meaning to, communicated to us that we were fat, unattractive, or simply not lovable. Sometimes, too, food may have been used as a form of love. As a result, either we try to quiet our anxiety with food, or we turn to food when we really need something else—a hug, a peaceful moment, an expression of appreciation. Our turning to sweet and starchy foods may also result from blood-sugar problems or from systemic candida, an overgrowth of yeast that can lead to sugar cravings. Low serotonin levels—involved in depression and sleep problems—may also lead to sugar cravings.

These patterns can be challenging to rewrite, but taking some time for ourselves—for what *we* feel like, what *we* want to do—can be the first step toward turning them around. That's what I told Annette, and that's what I'm telling you. Taking time for yourself might be the healthiest decision you ever make.

Go Organic

Since environmental toxins can add to your allostatic load and further stress your adrenals, one way to relieve some of that burden is to eat organic as much as possible. I know that can be challenging if you're not used to it and it can also be somewhat more expensive than eating so-called conventionally farmed foods. The healthy compromise might be to make just a few changes—going organic for the foods that are most likely to retain pesticides and eating the safer conventional foods.

Consider, too, that even after washing, some fruits and vegetables carry higher pesticide residues than others, according to the U.S. Department of Agriculture (USDA). Researchers at the Washington, D.C.–based advocacy organization, Environmental Working Group, analyzed more than 100,000 U.S. government pesticide test results and put together the following "dirty dozen" list: fruits and vegetables that, if grown conventionally or imported, are most likely to retain pesticides. If you're only going to make a few organic choices, these foods should be at the top of your list:

- Apples

- Bell peppers

- Celery

- Cherries

- Grapes

- Nectarines

- Peaches

- Pears

- Potatoes

- Raspberries

- Spinach

- Strawberries

By contrast, these conventionally grown products are less likely to retain pesticides:

- Asparagus

- Avocados

- Bananas

- Broccoli

- Cauliflower

- Corn

- Kiwi fruit

- Mangos

- Onions

- Papayas

- Peas

- Pineapples

Milk, beef, and poultry are also good choices for your organic list because of the antibiotics, growth hormones, and feed given to conventionally grown cows and chickens, and the problematic ways that these animals are raised. If you're buying conventional, at least discard the fatty parts—the poultry skin and beef fat—where pesticides and toxins tend to reside. You might also just look for grass-fed beef with no antibiotics. As always, make changes to the best of your ability, and don't stress out about it.

Be mindful of labels when you're buying seafood. The term "organic" can be applied to either wild or farmed fish, because no USDA certification standards exist for seafood. In other words, the label means whatever the manufacturer wants it to mean.

Use Healthy Sweeteners

If you would like to use a sweetener, I can recommend the following healthy choices: erythritol, xylitol, and stevia. Erythritol is a natural sugar alcohol found in fruits and fermented fruits. It does not affect blood sugar and does not contribute to tooth decay. It is 60 to 70 percent as sweet as table sugar yet it is almost noncaloric. Xylitol is found in the fibers of many fruits and vegetables, including various berries, corn husks, oats, and mushrooms. It is about as sweet as sucrose (table sugar) with only two-thirds of the calories. Stevia is an herbal supplement from the South American plant *Stevia rebaudiana*. It is a very sweet sugar substitute. (For more information on stevia, see https://nunaturals.com).

By the way, although agave syrup is very popular these days, I don't recommend it. According to many experts, it's actually worse than high-fructose corn syrup because it contains so much fructose, which is such an aggressive sweetener that it can cause all sorts of problems, including increased inflammation. This is true despite the fact that agave has a low glycemic index. So skip the agave syrup and make a healthier choice.

The 90–10 Rule

I believe in moderation in all things. Especially as you begin your new regimen, go easy on yourself! Allow yourself to shoot for only 90 percent compliance. The other 10 percent of what you eat is up to you.

If you're doing the math, that means out of 35 meals and snacks per week, 4 are your call. So 4 times a week, if you want to add something that feels like a special treat, feel free, as long as you don't consume any gluten or sugar, which will really slow your progress. However, if this feels too restrictive, just do the best you can. In any case, allow yourself to really savor whatever "extra" food you've chosen. Eat it slowly, in a comfortable place, so that you can fully enjoy your 10 percent. If you're going for treats, make the most of them!

WHAT'S IN A NAME?

Confused by what's on the label? You're not alone. Here are some quick definitions to help you make the best choices at the grocery store:

"Organic" means:

- Animals have not been treated with antibiotics, growth hormones, or feed made from animal by-products.

- Animals must have been given organic feed for at least a year.

- Animals must have access to the outdoors.

- Food hasn't been genetically modified or irradiated.

- Fertilizer does not contain sewage sludge or synthetic ingredients.

- Produce hasn't been contaminated with synthetic chemicals used as pesticides.

Label definitions:

- "100% Organic": Product must contain 100 percent organic ingredients.

- "Organic": At least 95 percent of ingredients are organically produced.

- "Made with Organic Ingredients": At least 70 percent of ingredients are organic. The remaining 30 percent must come from a list of particular products approved by the USDA.

- "Free-range" or "Free-roaming": Misleading term applied to chicken, eggs, and meat, since outdoor access must only be made available for "an undetermined period each day." In other words, don't assume that the animal spent a significant portion of its life outdoors.

- "Natural" or "All Natural": Don't confuse this term with organic, because this term has no standard definition except for meat and poultry. In that case, the USDA defines "natural" as not containing any artificial flavorings, colors, chemical preservatives, or synthetic ingredients. Otherwise, it's just a marketing term.

Listening to Your Body

Although it took Annette a couple of weeks to get used to the adrenal-friendly eating plan, she came to really enjoy her new approach to food. She liked eating "all day long" with her new regimen of three meals and two snacks. She was relieved to have a constant, steady flow of energy, thanks to her steady blood sugar, her adrenal supplements, and her avoidance of caffeine and sugar highs and lows. She found herself losing weight easily, which pleased her. But most important, she told me she felt that, for the first time in a long while, she was listening to her body, hearing what it needed and responding to that need.

"I hadn't realized I'd gotten so out of touch with myself," she said on her last visit. "If I was tired, I'd just grab another cup of coffee or a muffin. If I felt foggy, I'd grab a soda. If I was wired at the end of the night, I'd calm down with a bedtime snack. I just wasn't paying attention to how tired I was and how depleted I felt. I wasn't figuring out what I *really* needed."

I knew just what Annette meant. So often, when our body is craving, say, spinach, we know we're hungry for *something*. But if we reach for the foods we're most used to, we might end up eating two or three times as much as we need to, trying to satisfy a craving for something else. And if what we're *really* hungry for is a hug or a kind word, we'll eat quite a bit more than we need to, because the satisfaction won't really come from the food.

I'd like to end this chapter by sharing with you parts of an e-mail I received in response to the publication of *The Core Balance Diet,* my earlier book on food and health. I was so moved to hear from someone who seemed to be doing all the right things—exercising, restricting calories—but who couldn't lose weight until she allowed herself to slow down, take care of herself, and listen to her body:

I am writing you to thank you for your CORE BALANCE diet. First of all, I should tell you my short history. I am a physical therapist, certified Pilates instructor, and have authored two fitness books. I have worked with women in fitness for 25 years. I hear all their stories and frustrations on weight loss and diet. For the past four years I have gradually put on 20 pounds. I know about calories, I know about exercise. I practiced cardiac rehab for ten years. DIET I know. But I could not figure out what my problem was. I saw an endocrinologist, a dietician, an ob/gyn, my trainer, went to Weight Watchers, etc., and no one could explain to me what was going on. AND I could not lose weight. I just kept losing and gaining the same 5 pounds. All I kept hearing is that you are in perimenopause (I am 47) and this is normal. Just eat less and exercise more. I knew in my heart that this was wrong. I know my body.

I had been following your website for a few years and finally saw your book. I read it and it described me to a T. I am now on week three and have already lost 10 pounds. I have not seen the scale move in four years. I feel great, too. Like I said, exercise is my life and job. I teach four classes a week and also do my own fitness program on four days (Jazzercise, yoga, Pilates, and biking). I knew it was not my activity level. When they told me to exercise more, I was just more tired and did not lose any weight. I know now that I needed to back off a bit and let my adrenals heal—since I scored very high on that test.

Anyway, thank you for your wonderful book. . . . I LOVE the recipes and so does my family. This has been a win-win all the way around. You have my utmost respect for listening, research-ing, and not dismissing our problems as women. . . .

If someone who teaches exercise can benefit from slowing down and caring for herself, what better testimony could there be? I invite you to listen to your body the way Annette and this reader listened to theirs. As the reader said in her e-mail, that can only be a "win-win."

chapter six

YOUR 30-DAY ADRENAL-FRIENDLY EATING PLAN

So here it is: your 30-day adrenal-friendly eating plan. As you can see, it includes three meals and two snacks a day to keep your blood sugar nice and level, which will help prevent stress on your adrenals. These delicious dishes are easy to prepare and designed to satisfy both your hunger and your cravings for tasty food.

I have provided you with an eating plan, the recipes you need to follow the plan, and the shopping lists you can use to keep your kitchen well stocked. And for those of you who are vegetarians, you can find some alternate recipes later in this chapter.

I have designed the eating plan to give you maximum flexibility, so you can choose the foods that you like, that your family likes, and that you can easily find. In some cases, I've just put "fruit," which means you can choose any fruit from the "Adrenal-Friendly Pantry" on page 160. If I haven't given a portion size, feel free to eat as much of the item as you like—though if you're concerned about weight, I suggest you eat slowly, start with a smaller amount, pause for a little while after finishing your first portion, and give yourself a chance to feel full before going back for seconds.

Likewise, if you would like to substitute a different type of fruit, vegetable, or protein, feel free to go back to the adrenal-friendly pantry, and, for example, substitute blueberries or apples for strawberries. Feel free to switch out cashew butter for almond butter and vice versa. And if you want to switch out your proteins, here is the formula:

- You can substitute fish for eggs, chicken, turkey, or beef.

- You can substitute eggs, chicken, or turkey for fish.

However, don't eat any one type of food more than once a day, because your body can develop sensitivities when overexposed to a single food. Generally speaking, it's good for your body to have as wide a range of foods as possible, to get as many different types of nutrients as you can. But, as always, take it slow and do what feels right.

Finally, if you would like to eat less meat, you have the option of making a switch once or twice a week by substituting a vegetarian recipe (see page 147) for any of the protein dishes in the menu plan. Likewise, you're free to use the 90–10 rule to add an occasional adrenal-friendly treat (see page 96).

As you follow this diet, you will find yourself feeling better and perhaps even losing some weight. You will also be able to enjoy delicious food that satisfies your hunger and is a pleasure to eat. Enjoy!

Thirty Days to Adrenal Health

Recipes for items marked with an asterisk (*) can be found in the section on page 111.

DAY 1

Breakfast

Farm Fresh Omelet*
½ cup fresh fruit

Snack

½ cup unsweetened
Greek-style yogurt with
½ cup strawberries and
1 tablespoon crushed pecans

Sweeten your yogurt with
erythritol, stevia, or xylitol

Lunch

Tasty Turkey Cutlets*
1 cup mixed greens with
1 teaspoon olive oil and
juice of ½ lemon
1 small or ½ large
gluten-free roll

Snack

Three Cheese Dip* with cut-
up vegetables or spread on
large romaine lettuce leaves

Dinner

Marinated Shrimp
with Artichoke Hearts*
steamed broccoli
½ cup brown rice,
millet, or quinoa

DAY 2

Breakfast

Spinach Cups*
½ cup fresh berries

Snack

½ apple with 1 tablespoon
cashew butter

Lunch

leftover Marinated Shrimp
with Artichoke Hearts*
1 small or ½ large
gluten-free roll

Snack

Creamy Guacamole*
with cut-up vegetables

Dinner

chicken with 1 serving
Strawberry Salsa*
1 cup mixed greens
with 1 teaspoon olive oil
and juice of ½ lemon
½ cup brown rice, millet,
or quinoa

DAY 3

Breakfast

Tempting Turkey Hash*
melon wedge (honeydew
or cantaloupe) or ½ cup
raspberries

Snack

½ cup unsweetened Greek-
style yogurt with
½ cup berries

Lunch

Italian Chicken Soup*
2 large or 4 small
gluten-free crackers

Snack

Swiss Stacker*

Dinner

broiled salmon
Sautéed Kale*
½ cup brown rice,
millet, or quinoa

DAY 4

Breakfast

Easy Feta Omelet*
½ cup fresh berries

Snack

½ apple stuffed with
2 tablespoons ricotta cheese
and topped with cinnamon
and 1 tablespoon
chopped nuts

Lunch

leftover salmon with
Minty Yogurt Sauce*
1 cup mixed greens with
1 teaspoon olive oil and
juice of ½ lemon
1 small or ½ large
gluten-free roll

Snack

2 tablespoons hummus
with vegetables

Dinner

Pork with Tomato
Cream Sauce*
Cajun Rice*
steamed kale

DAY 5

Breakfast
Salmon Patties*
½ cup unsweetened Greek-style yogurt with
½ cup berries

Snack
½ apple with 1 tablespoon cashew butter

Lunch
leftover Pork with
Tomato Cream Sauce* on
bed of 1 cup mixed greens
1 small or ½ large
gluten-free roll

Snack
Three Cheese Dip* with cut-up vegetables or spread on large romaine lettuce leaves

Dinner
Aromatic Apple Chicken*
1 cup mixed greens with
1 teaspoon olive oil and
juice of ½ lemon
½ cup brown rice,
millet, or quinoa

DAY 6

Breakfast
Cheesy Eggs*

Snack
½ cup unsweetened
Greek-style yogurt with
½ cup strawberries and
1 tablespoon crushed nuts

Lunch
Quick Turkey Stir-fry*
½ cup brown rice,
millet, or quinoa

Snack
Swiss Stacker*

Dinner
Easy Lamb Chops*
Parmesan Asparagus*
½ baked sweet potato with
½ teaspoon butter; sprinkle
with cinnamon if desired

DAY 7

Breakfast
Asparagus Frittata*

Snack
Easiest-Ever
Strawberry smoothie*

Lunch
Tasty Turkey Cutlets*
steamed spinach
1 small or ½ large
gluten-free roll

Snack
½ apple with almond butter

Dinner
Lentil Casserole*
1 cup mixed greens with
1 teaspoon olive oil and
juice of ½ lemon

DAY 8

Breakfast
Homemade Turkey Patties*
½ cup unsweetened Greek-style yogurt with fruit

Snack
Dilly Devils*

Lunch
Italian Chicken Soup*
1 cup mixed greens with
1 teaspoon olive oil and
juice of ½ lemon
1 small or ½ large
gluten-free roll

Snack
2 tablespoons hummus
with vegetables

Dinner
Garden-Inspired Baked
Haddock* ½ cup brown rice,
millet, or quinoa

DAY 9

Breakfast
Easy Feta Omelet*

Snack
½ apple and 1 tablespoon almond butter

Lunch
leftover Lentil Casserole*

Snack
Turkey Poppers*

Dinner
Easy Lamb Chops*
½ cup steamed vegetables
½ baked sweet potato with
½ teaspoon butter; sprinkle
with cinnamon if desired

DAY 10

Breakfast
½ cup unsweetened
Greek-style yogurt with
½ cup strawberries and 2
tablespoons crushed pecans

Snack
½ apple stuffed with 2
tablespoons ricotta cheese
and topped with cinnamon

and 1 tablespoon
chopped nuts

Lunch
Waldorf Turkey Salad*
over 1 cup mixed greens
with 1 teaspoon olive oil
and juice of ½ lemon
1 small or ½ large
gluten-free roll

Snack
Salmon Roll-up*

Dinner
Easy Chicken Stir-fry*
½ cup brown rice,
millet, or quinoa

DAY 11

Breakfast
Savory Artichoke Squares*
melon wedge (honeydew or
cantaloupe) or ½ cup berries

Snack
½ cup unsweetened
Greek-style yogurt with
½ cup strawberries and 1
tablespoon crushed pecans

Lunch
Spicy Shrimp and
Brown Rice*
1 cup mixed greens with
1 teaspoon olive oil and
juice of ½ lemon

Snack
Three Cheese Dip* with cut-
up vegetables or spread on
large romaine lettuce leaves

Dinner
JASS-Y Salad*
1 small or ½ large
gluten-free roll

DAY 12

Breakfast
Homemade
Turkey Patties*
2 eggs, any style
melon wedge (honeydew
or cantaloupe) or
½ cup berries

Snack
Orange Ricotta Dream*

Lunch
leftover JASS-Y Salad*
1 small or ½ large
gluten-free roll

Snack
Three Cheese Dip* with cut-
up vegetables or spread on
large romaine lettuce leaves

Dinner
Turkey Creole*
½ cup brown rice,
millet, or quinoa
Creamy Cucumber Salad*

DAY 13

Breakfast
Tempting Turkey Hash*
½ cup raspberries

Snack
½ apple with
1 tablespoon
cashew butter

Lunch
Speedy Beef Stir-fry*
1 small or ½ large
gluten-free roll

Snack
½ cup unsweetened
Greek-style yogurt with
½ cup strawberries and 1
tablespoon crushed nuts

Dinner
chicken—grilled or roasted
Roasted Brussels Sprouts*
½ cup brown rice,
millet, or quinoa

DAY 14

Breakfast
Spinach Cups*
½ cup fresh berries

Snack
Salmon Roll-up*

Lunch
Tasty Turkey Cutlets*
steamed broccoli
1 small or ½ large
gluten-free roll

Snack
2 tablespoons hummus
with vegetables

Dinner
Mary's Stuffed Chicken*
1 cup mixed greens with
1 teaspoon olive oil and juice
of ½ lemon
½ baked sweet potato with
½ teaspoon butter; sprinkle
with cinnamon if desired

DAY 15

Breakfast
Homemade Turkey Patties*
½ cup unsweetened Greek-
style yogurt with ½ cup fruit
Sweeten your yogurt with
erythritol, stevia, or xylitol

Snack
½ apple stuffed with ricotta
cheese and topped with
cinnamon and chopped nuts

Lunch
leftover Mary's Stuffed
Chicken* on 1 small or
½ large gluten-free roll
Zucchini Soup*

Snack
Swiss Stacker*

Dinner
Crab Cakes*
Curried Rice*
steamed broccoli

DAY 16

Breakfast
Cheesy Eggs*
1 slice gluten-free toast
with 1 tablespoon
all-fruit/no-sugar
fruit spread

Snack
Easiest-Ever Strawberry
Smoothie*

Lunch
leftover Crab Cakes*
leftover Curried Rice*
1 cup mixed greens with
1 teaspoon olive oil and juice
of ½ lemon

Snack
Turkey Poppers*

Dinner
Easy Lamb Chops*
½ cup brown rice, millet, or
quinoa
steamed asparagus

DAY 17

Breakfast
Tempting Turkey Hash*
½ cup fruit

Snack
½ apple stuffed with
2 tablespoons ricotta
cheese and topped with
cinnamon and 1 tablespoon
chopped nuts

Lunch
Waldorf Turkey Salad*
over 1 cup mixed greens
with 1 teaspoon olive oil
and juice of ½ lemon
1 small or ½ large
gluten-free roll

Snack
Three Cheese Dip* with cut-
up vegetables or spread on
large romaine lettuce leaves

Dinner
California Chicken*
Twisted Cauliflower*
½ baked sweet potato with
½ teaspoon butter; sprinkle
with cinnamon if desired

DAY 18

Breakfast
½ cup unsweetened
Greek-style yogurt with
½ cup blueberries and
2 tablespoons crushed
pecans

Snack
Dilly Devils*

Lunch
Easy Chicken Stir-fry*

Snack
Salmon Roll-up*

Dinner
Donna's Favorite Haddock*
Ginger-y Brussels Sprouts*
1 cup mixed greens with
1 teaspoon olive oil and
juice of ½ lemon
½ cup brown rice,
millet, or quinoa

DAY 19

Breakfast
Easy Feta Omelet*
melon wedge (honeydew
or cantaloupe) or
½ cup berries

Snack
½ cup unsweetened Greek-
style yogurt with ½ apple
cut into wedges

Lunch
Spicy Crab Salad * over
1 cup mixed greens with
1 teaspoon olive oil and
juice of ½ lemon
1 small or ½ large
gluten-free roll

Snack
2 tablespoons hummus
with vegetables

Dinner
baked chicken breast
Tomato-Topped Zucchini*
½ baked sweet potato with
½ teaspoon butter; sprinkle
with cinnamon if desired

DAY 20

Breakfast
2 eggs, any style
1 slice gluten-free toast
with 1 tablespoon
all-fruit/no-sugar fruit spread
melon wedge (honeydew
or cantaloupe) or
½ cup berries

Snack
½ apple with 1 tablespoon
cashew butter

Lunch
Spicy Shrimp and
Brown Rice*
1 cup mixed greens with
1 teaspoon olive oil and
juice of ½ lemon

Snack
Swiss Stacker*

Dinner
broiled or baked turkey
cutlets with Pesto*
1 cup mixed greens with
1 teaspoon olive oil and
juice of ½ lemon
½ cup brown rice,
millet, or quinoa

DAY 21

Breakfast
Tempting Turkey Hash*
½ cup raspberries

Snack
½ cup unsweetened Greek-style yogurt with ½ cup berries and 1 tablespoon crushed pecans

Lunch
Crab-Stuffed Avocado*
2 large or 4 small gluten-free crackers

Snack
Three Cheese Dip* with cut-up vegetables or spread on large romaine lettuce leaves

Dinner
Easy Chicken Stir-fry*
½ cup brown rice, millet, or quinoa

DAY 22

Breakfast
½ cup unsweetened Greek-style yogurt with ½ cup mixed berries
1 slice gluten-free toast with 1 tablespoon almond butter

Snack
½ apple stuffed with 2 tablespoons ricotta cheese and topped with cinnamon

and 1 tablespoon chopped nuts

Lunch
Italian Chicken Soup*
2 large or 4 small gluten-free crackers
melon wedge (honeydew or cantaloupe) or ½ cup berries

Snack
Creamy Guacamole* with cut-up vegetables

Dinner
Marinated Shrimp with Artichoke Hearts*
1 cup mixed greens with 1 teaspoon olive oil and juice of ½ lemon ½ cup brown rice, millet, or quinoa

DAY 23

Breakfast
Homemade Turkey Patties*
Sweet-Potato Hash*
¼ cup berries

Snack
½ apple with 1 tablespoon cashew butter

Lunch
broiled or baked chicken on mixed greens
2 large or 4 small gluten-free crackers
melon wedge (honeydew or cantaloupe) or ½ cup berries

Snack
Salmon Roll-up*

Dinner
Speedy Beef Stir-fry*
½ cup brown rice, millet, or quinoa

DAY 24

Breakfast
Spinach Cups*
1 slice gluten-free toast with 1 tablespoon nut butter

Snack
Easy Turkey Roll-ups*

Lunch
leftover Marinated Shrimp with Artichoke Hearts*
1 cup mixed greens with 1 teaspoon olive oil and juice of ½ lemon
1 small or ½ large gluten-free roll

Snack
Swiss Stacker*

Dinner
Donna's Favorite Haddock*
steamed broccoli
½ baked sweet potato with ½ teaspoon butter; sprinkle with cinnamon if desired

DAY 25

Breakfast

2-egg omelet—vegetables
plus 1 ounce any cheese
½ cup berries
1 slice gluten-free toast with
1 tablespoon cashew butter

Snack

Easiest-Ever Strawberry
Smoothie*

Lunch

Waldorf Turkey Salad*
2 large or 4 small
gluten-free crackers

Snack

Three Cheese Dip* with cut-
up vegetables or spread on
large romaine lettuce leaves

Dinner

Easy Lamb Chops*
steamed spinach
½ baked sweet potato with
½ teaspoon butter; sprinkle
with cinnamon if desired

DAY 26

Breakfast

Salmon Patties*
½ cup berries

Snack

½ apple with
1 tablespoon
almond butter

Lunch

broiled or grilled steak
Sautéed Kale*
1 small or ½ large
gluten-free roll

Snack

Three Cheese Dip* with cut-
up vegetables or spread on
large romaine lettuce leaves

Dinner

Cilantro-Lime Shrimp*
½ cup steamed pea pods
½ cup brown rice,
millet, or quinoa

DAY 27

Breakfast

½ cup unsweetened
Greek-style yogurt with
½ cup berries and
1 tablespoons nuts
1 slice gluten-free bread with
1 tablespoon
cashew butter

Snack

Easiest-Ever Strawberry
Smoothie*

Lunch

Tasty Ten-Minute Chicken*
1 cup mixed greens with
1 teaspoon olive oil and
juice of ½ lemon
1 small or ½ large
gluten-free roll

Snack

Turkey Poppers*

Dinner

Aromatic Apple Chicken*
Parmesan Asparagus*
½ baked sweet potato with
½ teaspoon butter; sprinkle
with cinnamon if desired

DAY 28

Breakfast

Tempting Turkey Hash*
½ cup berries

Snack

½ apple stuffed with
2 tablespoons ricotta
cheese and topped with
cinnamon and 1 tablespoon
chopped nuts

Lunch

Italian Chicken Soup*
2 large or 4 small
gluten-free crackers

Snack

Swiss Stacker*

Dinner

Salmon Surprise*
steamed spinach
½ cup brown rice,
millet, or quinoa

DAY 29

Breakfast

Asparagus Frittata*
melon wedge (honeydew
or cantaloupe) or
½ cup berries

Snack

½ cup unsweetened Greek-
style yogurt with ½ cup
berries

Lunch

Spicy Crab Salad*
1 small or ½ large
gluten-free roll

Snack

2 tablespoons hummus
with vegetables

Dinner

Tasty Turkey Cutlets*
steamed broccoli
½ baked sweet potato with
½ teaspoon butter; sprinkle
with cinnamon if desired

DAY 30

Breakfast

Homemade Turkey Patties*
½ cup unsweetened Greek-
style yogurt with ½ cup
berries

Snack

Dilly Devils*

Lunch

Tasty Ten-Minute
Chicken*
½ cup brown rice,
millet, or quinoa

Snack

Easy Turkey Roll-ups*

Dinner

Crab-Stuffed Avocado*
½ cup brown rice,
millet, or quinoa

Recipes

Here are the recipes you'll need to follow your 30-day eating plan. There's a list of vegetarian recipes, too, which you can use to substitute for the ones that rely on meat, poultry, or seafood as the main ingredient.

AROMATIC APPLE CHICKEN

1 teaspoon olive oil
2 boneless skinless chicken breasts
Salt and pepper to taste
½ cup thinly sliced Granny Smith apples
½ medium shallot, thinly sliced
½ tablespoon fresh thyme leaves
3 tablespoons balsamic vinegar

Preheat oven to 375 degrees.

Lightly oil shallow baking dish. Place chicken in baking dish and season with salt and pepper.

Arrange apple slices, shallots, and thyme leaves over and around chicken breasts. Pour balsamic vinegar over all.

Bake for 15 to 20 minutes, or until chicken is cooked through. Serve.

2 servings

ASPARAGUS FRITTATA

1 teaspoon olive oil
½ yellow onion, finely chopped
½ pound asparagus, cut into small pieces
Salt and pepper to taste
4 eggs, beaten
½ cup shredded Swiss cheese

Preheat broiler. Wrap skillet handle in foil if not oven-proof.

In large skillet, heat olive oil over medium heat. Add onion and cook until translucent.

Add asparagus, salt, and pepper, and cook until desired tenderness is reached.

Pour eggs over asparagus and onions. Cook until mixture is almost set.

Sprinkle cheese on frittata. Then place skillet under broiler until cheese is hot and bubbly. Watch closely. Do not allow cheese to brown. Serve.

Note: Use oven mitts to carefully remove hot skillet from oven.

2 servings

CAJUN RICE

1 cup vegetable or chicken broth
1½ teaspoons Cajun seasoning
1 cup brown rice
2 cups kale, washed, stems removed, and torn into small pieces

In large pot, bring broth and Cajun seasoning to boil.

Stir in rice and kale and return to boil. Cover and reduce heat to low.

Cook approximately 30 to 40 minutes, or until all liquid is absorbed. Serve.

4 servings

CALIFORNIA CHICKEN

2 boneless skinless chicken breasts

1 avocado, peeled, pitted, and diced

½ medium tomato, seeds removed and diced

½ clove garlic, minced

2 tablespoons diced onion

2 tablespoons chopped cilantro

1½ tablespoons lime juice

1 tablespoon olive oil, for baking dish

Preheat oven to 350 degrees.

Slice a pocket in the thickest part of each chicken breast.

Mix remaining ingredients in bowl, reserving half of mixture. Spoon avocado mixture into chicken pocket and press opening closed, using toothpicks if necessary. Lightly oil shallow baking dish. Bake for approximately 40 minutes, or until chicken is cooked through. Serve with reserved avocado mixture.

2 servings

CHEESY EGGS

2 tablespoons ricotta cheese

1 tablespoon shredded Parmesan cheese

½ teaspoon olive oil

2 eggs, beaten

Salt and pepper to taste

In small bowl, combine cheeses.

Heat olive oil in small skillet over medium heat. Add eggs. Lift edges of egg mixture as it cooks to allow uncooked mixture to move to bottom of pan. When center is almost set, add cheese mixture, and salt and pepper. Fold in half using spatula and serve.

1 serving

CILANTRO-LIME SHRIMP

¾ pound shrimp, peeled and deveined
Juice from 1 lime
1 clove garlic, minced
1 tablespoon grated fresh ginger
1 tablespoon olive oil
2 tablespoons chopped cilantro
½ teaspoon grated lemon zest
Salt and pepper to taste

In large bowl, combine shrimp, lime juice, garlic, and ginger. Stir well.

In large skillet, heat olive oil over medium heat. Add shrimp mixture, and sauté approximately 5 minutes, or until shrimp are pink and cooked through. Remove pan from heat. Stir in cilantro and lemon zest. Season with salt and pepper, and serve.

2 servings

CRAB CAKES

1 cup gluten-free bread crumbs, plus extra for dredging
¼ teaspoon dry mustard
1½ tablespoons heavy cream
1 teaspoon lemon juice
Old Bay seasoning to taste
Pepper to taste
1 cup lump crabmeat
1 tablespoon olive oil, for skillet

In large bowl, mix all ingredients except crabmeat until well blended. Add crabmeat and mix well. Form into four patties approximately ½-inch thick. Lightly dredge patties in additional bread crumbs.

Heat olive oil in large skillet over medium heat. Cook patties for 2 minutes per side, or until lightly browned and heated through.

2 servings; 2 patties per serving

CRAB-STUFFED AVOCADO

6 ounces fresh crabmeat

½ cup chopped celery

3 tablespoons plain yogurt

1 teaspoon freshly squeezed lemon juice

Salt and pepper to taste

⅛ teaspoon paprika

1 ripe avocado, cut in half and pitted

In medium bowl, combine all ingredients except avocado. Mix well.

Spoon half of crab mixture into each avocado half.

2 servings

CREAMY CUCUMBER SALAD

2 medium cucumbers, peeled and thinly sliced

Salt and pepper to taste

4 tablespoons Greek-style yogurt

1 teaspoon red wine vinegar

2 tablespoons onion, minced

1 tablespoon chopped dill

In colander, generously salt cucumber slices and let drain approximately 1 hour.

In large bowl, combine remaining ingredients and mix well.

Add cucumbers. Add salt and pepper, and serve.

4 servings

CREAMY GUACAMOLE

½ ripe medium-sized avocado, peeled, pitted, and chopped
4 tablespoons sour cream
1 tablespoon chopped green chilies
Juice of ½ lemon

Chop avocado and place in small bowl and prepare to desired consistency.

- For creamy guacamole, mash with backside of fork. Add remaining ingredients and mix well.

- For smooth guacamole, process all ingredients in blender or food processor.

Keep refrigerated until ready to serve.

2 servings

CURRIED RICE

½ tablespoon olive oil
¼ cup finely chopped onion
½ clove garlic, minced
½ teaspoon curry powder, or more to taste
½ cup brown rice
1 cup chicken broth
2 tablespoons finely chopped Granny Smith apple
¼ cup walnuts

In large saucepan, heat oil over medium heat. Add onion and garlic, and cook until onion is translucent.

Add curry powder and stir well. Add rice and broth and bring to boil.

Reduce heat to low and cover. Cook 20 to 30 minutes, or until all liquid has been absorbed.

Add apple and nuts. Stir well and serve.

2 servings

DILLY DEVILS

¼ cup shredded cucumber

½ teaspoon salt

3 hard-cooked eggs

2 tablespoons Greek-style yogurt

1 tablespoon chopped dill

In small bowl, toss cucumber and salt and mix until well combined. Set aside.

Slice eggs in half. (Have fun and cut them in half crosswise!) Remove yolks and, in small bowl, mash yolks with back of fork. Set aside egg-white halves.

Add yogurt and dill to yolks.

Place cucumber mixture on towel and gently press out extra moisture. Combine with yogurt mixture.

Fill egg-white halves with 1 well-rounded teaspoon of mixture. Serve.

2 servings; 3 egg-white halves for each serving

DONNA'S FAVORITE HADDOCK

½ pound haddock
1 teaspoon olive oil, plus extra for baking dish
½ small onion, diced
1 clove garlic, minced
Salt and pepper to taste
½ cup ricotta cheese
1 egg, beaten
1 plum tomato, sliced
½ cup shredded mozzarella cheese

Preheat oven to 350 degrees.

Cut haddock into two pieces. Set aside.

In medium skillet, heat oil over medium heat. Add onion and garlic, and sauté until onion is soft and translucent. Add salt and pepper. Remove skillet from heat and let cool for 10 minutes, then add ricotta and egg and mix well.

Lightly oil shallow baking dish. Create two separate mounds of ricotta cheese mixture.

Lay piece of haddock over each mound of ricotta.

Bake uncovered for 8 minutes. Remove baking dish from oven and top each piece of haddock with two slices tomato and ¼ cup mozzarella.

Return to oven and bake 3 to 4 minutes longer, or until haddock is cooked through. Serve.

2 servings

EASIEST-EVER STRAWBERRY SMOOTHIE

7 large or 10 medium fresh strawberries

½ cup Greek-style yogurt

1 scoop whey or soy protein powder (Use the scoop that comes with the powder.)

½ cup ice cubes

Place all ingredients in blender and mix to desired consistency. Serve in a glass.

1 serving

EASY CHICKEN STIR-FRY

1 tablespoon olive oil

½ medium onion, chopped

1 large boneless skinless chicken breast, about 6 ounces, cut into cubes

2 cups fresh spinach, washed and stems removed

2 ounces fresh mushrooms, washed and sliced

1 tablespoon gluten-free soy sauce

1 cup cooked brown rice

In large skillet, heat the olive oil over medium heat. Add onion, stirring occasionally until translucent. Add chicken and stir until chicken is no longer pink and juices run clear. Add spinach and mushrooms. Stir and continue cooking until vegetables reach desired doneness. Add soy sauce and stir well. Serve over ½ cup brown rice.

2 servings

EASY FETA OMELET

¼ teaspoon olive oil
½ cup torn fresh spinach leaves
1 egg, beaten
1 tablespoon crumbled feta
½ medium tomato, diced
3 Kalamata olives, chopped

In small skillet, heat oil over medium heat.

In small bowl, mix spinach leaves with beaten egg. Pour egg mixture in pan and cook 2 to 3 minutes, or just until egg starts to set. Reduce heat to low, crumble cheese over egg, and cook approximately 2 minutes. Top with tomato and olives. Gently fold omelet in half and serve.

1 serving

EASY LAMB CHOPS

2 loin lamb chops
½ cup chopped onion
1 tablespoon dried mustard
3 tablespoons shredded Parmesan cheese
3 tablespoons unsweetened Greek-style yogurt

Preheat oven to 425 degrees.

Place chops on roasting rack in pan.

In medium bowl, mix remaining ingredients and spread evenly over chops.

Bake approximately 40 minutes, or until lamb reaches desired doneness. Serve.

2 servings

EASY TURKEY ROLL-UPS

4 tablespoons cream cheese

1 tablespoon chopped green onion

¼ cup chopped spinach leaves

2 slices oven-roasted deli turkey

Mix cream cheese, green onion, and spinach together. Spread evenly over turkey slices.

Roll each slice tightly and serve.

1 serving

FARM FRESH OMELET

4 eggs

Salt and pepper to taste

1 tablespoon butter

½ small onion, chopped

¼ cup chopped green pepper

½ small zucchini, chopped

⅓ cup shredded Swiss cheese

3 tablespoons heavy cream

½ cup chopped tomato

Pinch dried oregano

In small bowl, beat eggs. Add salt and pepper.

In medium pan over medium heat, melt butter, then add onion, green pepper, and zucchini. Sauté until vegetables reach desired tenderness. Remove from pan. Increasing heat to medium-high, pour egg mixture into pan. Lift cooked edges to allow uncooked eggs to move to bottom. When last of mixture shifts to bottom of pan, reduce heat to low. Add cheese, cream, cooked vegetables, tomato, and oregano. Fold egg mixture over in half. Continue cooking until cheese melts and vegetables are heated through. Serve.

2 servings

GARDEN-INSPIRED BAKED HADDOCK

½ pound haddock
1 tablespoon olive oil
1 clove garlic, minced
½ onion, finely chopped
½ green pepper, chopped
1 medium tomato, diced
2 tablespoons chopped fresh basil
2 teaspoons lemon juice

Preheat oven to 375 degrees.

Wash haddock and pat dry. Set aside.

In large skillet, heat oil over medium heat. Sauté garlic and onion until tender. Add green pepper, then reduce heat. Sauté over low heat until peppers reach desired tenderness. Add tomato and basil, stirring gently to combine all ingredients.

Place half of vegetable mixture in bottom of 8 x 8 baking dish.

Place haddock on top of vegetable mixture and top with remaining vegetable mixture. Drizzle with lemon juice. Cover and bake for 15 minutes, or until fish flakes easily. Serve.

2 servings

GINGER-Y BRUSSELS SPROUTS

1 cup Brussels sprouts

⅔ cup water

½ tablespoon gluten-free soy sauce

1 tablespoon minced fresh ginger

1 clove garlic, minced

Red pepper flakes to taste

Wash Brussels sprouts. Remove outer leaves and trim bottoms if needed. Drain well and set aside.

Place remaining ingredients in large saucepan over medium-high heat and bring to boil. Reduce heat to low and simmer for 4 minutes. Add Brussels sprouts and cover. Cook for 8 to 10 minutes, or until sprouts reach desired tenderness.

2 servings

HOMEMADE TURKEY PATTIES (ADAPTED FROM *THE CORE BALANCE DIET*)

1 pound ground turkey

4 egg whites

¼ cup minced green onion

⅔ cup dried parsley

⅜ teaspoon dried marjoram

Salt and pepper to taste

½ tablespoon olive oil

In medium bowl, crumble turkey. Mix in egg whites, green onion, parsley, and marjoram. Add salt and pepper. Shape turkey mixture into 12 small patties.

In large skillet, heat olive oil over medium to medium-high heat. Cook for 5 to 6 minutes on each side, or until patties are cooked through. Serve.

Refrigerate or freeze leftovers.

6 servings; 2 patties per serving

ITALIAN CHICKEN SOUP

One 14-ounce can low-sodium, gluten-free chicken broth
One 14.5-ounce can stewed tomatoes
1 clove garlic, minced
1 teaspoon dried basil
2 boneless skinless chicken breasts, cooked and chopped, about 1 cup
1½ cups chopped escarole
1½ tablespoons olive oil

In large saucepan over medium-high heat, bring chicken broth, tomatoes, garlic, and basil to a boil. Reduce heat to low and add chicken, escarole, and oil. Simmer for 10 minutes, and serve.

4 servings

JASS-Y SALAD (JÍCAMA, AVOCADO, SPINACH, AND SHRIMP)

1½ cups cooked shrimp
2 cups fresh spinach, washed and trimmed
½ ripe avocado, peeled, pitted, and cubed
½ medium jícama, diced
2 tablespoons olive oil
Juice from ½ lime
½ clove garlic, crushed
½ teaspoon chili powder
Salt and pepper to taste

To make the salad: In large bowl, toss together shrimp, spinach, avocado, and jícama.

To make the dressing: In small bowl, mix together olive oil, lime juice, garlic, chili powder, and salt and pepper. Drizzle dressing over salad and serve.

2 servings

LENTIL CASSEROLE

1 cup gluten-free chicken or vegetable broth
¼ cup lentils
¼ cup uncooked brown rice
1 clove garlic, minced
⅓ cup chopped onion
1 teaspoon oregano
1 teaspoon dried basil
⅓ cup grated Parmesan cheese

Preheat oven to 300 degrees.

Mix all ingredients except cheese in shallow baking dish. Cover and bake for 75 minutes. Remove cover, sprinkle with cheese, and bake additional 15 minutes, or until cheese is melted. Serve.

2 servings

MARINATED SHRIMP WITH ARTICHOKE HEARTS

1 pound uncooked shrimp, peeled and deveined
Two 7-ounce jars marinated artichoke hearts, reserving ⅓ cup marinade
2 large garlic cloves, coarsely chopped
½ cup olive oil, separated into two ¼ cups
2 tablespoons chopped fresh basil
Salt and pepper to taste

Preheat oven to 400 degrees.

In large bowl, combine shrimp, artichoke hearts and liquid, garlic, ¼ cup olive oil, 1 tablespoon basil, and salt and pepper. Mix well. Cover and marinate at least 20 minutes, stirring several times.

Remove shrimp from marinade and place in glass baking dish. Pour remaining olive oil and reserved artichoke marinade over shrimp. Cover tightly and bake 15 to 17 minutes, or until shrimp are pink and cooked.

Sprinkle with remaining basil and serve.

4 servings

MARY'S STUFFED CHICKEN

½ teaspoon olive oil, plus extra for baking dish
½ pound chopped fresh spinach
¼ cup part-skim ricotta cheese
¼ cup chopped onion
2 tablespoons grated Parmesan cheese
1 egg white, lightly beaten
2 boneless skinless chicken breasts, about 4 ounces each
1 tablespoon chicken broth

Preheat oven to 350 degrees.

Prepare 8 x 8 glass baking dish by lightly rubbing with olive oil.

In large bowl, combine spinach, ricotta, onion, cheese, and oil. Mix well. Reserve ½ cup mixture and set aside. Add egg white to remaining mixture.

Flatten chicken breasts to about ½-inch thick. Spread 2 tablespoons mixture over each chicken breast. Tightly roll up chicken breasts and press edges together, using toothpicks if necessary. Place in prepared pan, seam side down. Bake about 25 minutes, or until cooked through.

Put reserved spinach mixture and broth in a blender and process until smooth. Spoon over top of chicken and continue to cook for 5 more minutes. Serve.

2 servings

MINTY YOGURT SAUCE

2 heaping tablespoons chopped mint sprigs

½ large English cucumber, chopped

1½ cups unsweetened Greek-style yogurt

1 clove garlic, finely chopped

Salt and pepper to taste

In large bowl, combine all ingredients. Chill before serving.

4 servings

ORANGE RICOTTA DREAM

1 cup part-skim ricotta cheese

½ teaspoon grated orange zest

½ teaspoon freshly squeezed orange juice

½ teaspoon gluten-free vanilla extract

1½ teaspoons stevia

2 dashes cinnamon

In medium bowl, mix all ingredients together. Refrigerate for 1 hour.

If desired, top each serving with 1 tablespoon blueberries, strawberries, or raspberries.

2 servings

PARMESAN ASPARAGUS

½ pound thin asparagus spears
1½ teaspoons olive oil
3 tablespoons shaved Parmesan cheese
Freshly ground black pepper to taste
2 tablespoons balsamic vinegar

Preheat oven to 450 degrees.

In baking sheet, toss asparagus with olive oil, then arrange in single layer. Sprinkle cheese, then season with black pepper. Bake 12 to 14 minutes, or until cheese is melted and asparagus is tender-crisp. Sprinkle with balsamic vinegar and serve.

2 servings

PESTO

2 large cloves garlic
3½ cups fresh basil leaves, packed
½ cup olive oil, separated into two ¼ cups
½ cup pecans
¼ cup water
Salt to taste
¾ cup grated Parmesan cheese

Using a food processor, mince garlic, then add basil, ¼ cup olive oil, pecans, water, and salt. Puree until smooth, taking care to scrape down sides to ensure smooth mixture. Pour into bowl, then stir in cheese and remaining olive oil. Serve with turkey cutlets or other dish.

Note: Keeps well in covered container in refrigerator.

Approximately 8 servings; use to your own taste

PORK WITH TOMATO CREAM SAUCE

1 tablespoon plus 1 teaspoon olive oil
Two 4-ounce pork loin steaks
½ medium onion, chopped
1 clove garlic, finely chopped
1 plum tomato, seeded and chopped
1 tablespoon oregano
⅓ cup heavy cream
⅓ cup shredded Parmesan cheese

In large saucepan, heat 1 tablespoon oil over medium heat. Add pork steaks and cook 5 minutes per side, or until done. Remove pork from pan and set aside. Add remaining olive oil to pan and heat. Add onion and garlic, and cook until onion is translucent. Add tomato and oregano. Stir in cream and cheese until cheese melts. Spoon sauce over pork and serve.

2 servings

QUICK TURKEY STIR-FRY

½ tablespoon cornstarch

½ tablespoon chopped ginger

½ tablespoon Bragg Liquid Aminos or gluten-free soy sauce

¼ cup gluten-free chicken broth

½ tablespoon olive oil

¼ medium onion, thinly sliced

¼ medium red bell pepper, thinly sliced

½ cup broccoli

2 tablespoons cashews

1½ cups diced cooked turkey

In small bowl, combine cornstarch, ginger, soy sauce, and broth. Mix well.

In frying pan or wok, heat oil over high heat. Add onion and stir constantly for approximately 1 minute, or until onions are translucent. Add bell pepper, broccoli, and cashews, and continue stirring until vegetables reach desired crispness. Stir in turkey and ginger-soy sauce and continue cooking 4 to 6 minutes, or until sauce thickens and turkey is heated through, stirring constantly.

1 serving

ROASTED BRUSSELS SPROUTS

½ pound Brussels sprouts, washed and trimmed
1 tablespoon olive oil
Salt and pepper to taste

Preheat oven to 400 degrees.

In large bowl, combine ingredients until Brussels sprouts are well coated. Place vegetables on baking sheet, and place on center rack in oven. Roast for approximately 35 minutes, turning every 6 minutes, until Brussels sprouts are dark brown and tender. Serve over ½ cup brown rice, along with grilled or roasted chicken.

2 servings

SALMON PATTIES

6 ounces salmon, flaked
1 egg, beaten
½ small onion, diced
1 teaspoon lemon juice
½ teaspoon marjoram
1 to 2 teaspoons olive oil, for skillet

In large bowl, mix all ingredients (except olive oil) together, then divide into four equal portions. Form ½-inch-thick patty from each portion.

In large skillet, heat olive oil over medium heat. Cook patties 3 to 4 minutes per side, or until salmon is cooked through.

2 servings; 2 patties per serving

SALMON ROLL-UP

1 ounce cream cheese, softened
1 teaspoon fresh lemon juice
1 teaspoon capers (optional)
4 ounces cured salmon, or lox

In small bowl, combine cream cheese, lemon juice, and capers, if using. Spread over salmon. Roll up salmon and serve.

1 serving

SALMON SURPRISE

¾ cup water
¼ cup white wine
1 bay leaf
1½ tablespoons scallions, thinly sliced
1 pound fresh salmon
1 teaspoon olive oil
1 cup fresh spinach
¼ teaspoon ground nutmeg
⅓ cup shredded Parmesan cheese

In large skillet, heat water, wine, bay leaf, and scallions to a boil. Add salmon and return to boil. Cover, reduce heat to simmer, and cook for 6 to 8 minutes, or until fish flakes easily.

Drizzle olive oil on baking sheet. Remove fish from skillet and place on baking sheet. Set aside.

Remove bay leaf from liquid mixture. Add spinach to liquid mixture in skillet. Stir gently over low heat until spinach wilts. Season with nutmeg. Remove spinach and layer over salmon. Sprinkle with cheese. Broil for approximately 2 minutes, or until cheese is melted and lightly browned. Serve.

4 servings; approximately 4 ounces per serving

SAUTÉED KALE

1 tablespoon olive oil
1 clove garlic, minced
½ head kale, washed, trimmed, and cut into small pieces
½ cup vegetable broth
1½ tablespoons freshly squeezed lemon juice, or to taste
Salt and pepper to taste

In large sauté pan, heat olive oil over medium heat. Add garlic and cook for 3 minutes, or until garlic is lightly browned. Add kale, stirring constantly and cook for 2 more minutes. Add vegetable broth and cover. Simmer for 5 minutes, or until kale reaches desired tenderness. Add lemon juice, salt, and pepper. Serve.

Note: This dish freezes well.

3 to 4 servings

SAVORY ARTICHOKE SQUARES

1 tablespoon olive oil
One 7-ounce jar marinated artichoke hearts, marinade reserved
1 large clove garlic, minced
½ small onion, finely chopped
2 large eggs, beaten
1 cup shredded sharp cheddar cheese
2 tablespoons gluten-free bread crumbs
Salt and pepper to taste

Preheat oven to 325 degrees and lightly oil 11 x 7 loaf pan.

In small sauté pan, combine marinade from artichoke hearts, garlic, and onions. Sauté until onion is translucent. Set aside in medium bowl.

Chop artichoke hearts and add to onion mixture. Add eggs, cheese, bread crumbs, and salt and pepper. Place mixture in prepared loaf pan, and bake 23 to 27 minutes, or until mixture is firm. Cool and cut into 4 pieces.

Note: This dish freezes well.

4 servings

SPEEDY BEEF STIR-FRY

½ cup chicken broth

1 tablespoon gluten-free soy sauce

½ teaspoon cornstarch

2 tablespoons olive oil

½ pound round steak, cut into thin slabs

½ cup onion, diced

2 cups broccoli florets

½ cup water chestnuts

In small bowl, combine broth, soy sauce, and cornstarch. Set aside.

In large skillet, heat oil over medium-high heat. Add beef and brown on both sides. Remove beef from pan and set aside. Add onion and broccoli, stirring constantly, until onion is translucent and broccoli reaches desired tenderness. Add beef, broth mixture, and water chestnuts to skillet. Stir well and continue cooking over medium heat, stirring constantly, until liquids thicken and all ingredients are heated through. Serve.

2 servings

SPICY CRAB SALAD

    2 tablespoons fresh lemon juice
    ½ tablespoon olive oil
    ½ teaspoon hot sauce, or to taste
    ½ pound crabmeat, well drained
    ½ ripe avocado, peeled, pitted, and diced
    Salt and pepper to taste
    Mixed greens

In small bowl, combine lemon juice, olive oil, and hot sauce.

In separate small bowl, mix crabmeat and avocado together. Add lemon juice mixture, and gently combine. Add salt and pepper.

Serve over mixed greens.

2 servings

SPICY SHRIMP AND BROWN RICE

½ pound shrimp

1 tablespoon olive oil

½ medium red onion, diced

2 cloves garlic, minced

Salt to taste

1 cup broccoli florets

½ small jalapeño, poblano pepper, or chili pepper, seeded and chopped

1 tablespoon Worcestershire sauce

½ cup uncooked brown rice

1 cup water

Peel and clean shrimp. Set aside.

In large skillet, heat olive oil over medium heat. Add onion and garlic, sautéing until onion is translucent. Add remaining ingredients and bring to boil. Reduce heat to medium, cover skillet, and simmer for 30 minutes, or until rice is soft. Add shrimp, re-cover, and simmer for an additional 5 to 7 minutes, or until shrimp is cooked through. Serve.

2 servings

SPINACH CUPS

6 ounces fresh spinach
½ cup part-skim ricotta cheese
½ cup shredded Parmesan cheese
2 large eggs, beaten
1 clove garlic, minced
¼ teaspoon salt
Freshly ground pepper to taste
Unsalted butter, for greasing muffin cups

Preheat oven to 400 degrees.

Finely chop spinach, using food processor if preferred. Then in large bowl, mix ingredients together well.

Lightly grease 4 muffin cups. Divide mixture among the 4 cups. Bake 17 to 20 minutes, or until the spinach cups are set. Cool in pan for 5 minutes, then loosen cups by running butter knife along edges. Serve.

2 servings; 2 spinach cups per serving

STRAWBERRY SALSA

1 cup fresh strawberries, sliced

2 medium tomatoes, seeded and chopped

Jalapeño pepper to taste, seeded and minced

1 clove garlic, minced

1 lime, juiced

1 tablespoon olive oil

2 tablespoons fresh cilantro

In large bowl, combine all ingredients until well blended.

Cover and chill for 1 hour. Serve.

2 servings

SWEET-POTATO HASH

½ tablespoon olive oil

½ medium sweet potato, cooked and skin removed, cut into cubes

1 teaspoon heavy cream

Dash ground ginger

In small skillet, heat oil over medium-high heat.

In small bowl, combine remaining ingredients. Using spatula or back of fork to flatten potatoes, sauté 2 to 3 minutes on each side, or until mixture is lightly browned on both sides. Serve.

1 serving

SWISS STACKER

1 tablespoon olive oil
Juice from ½ lemon
Salt and pepper to taste
1 medium tomato, sliced into 4 thick slices
1 ounce Swiss cheese, cut into 2 slices
1 teaspoon chopped basil
2 slices cucumber
1 slice Vidalia onion, separated into 4 rings

To make dressing: in small bowl, combine oil, lemon juice, and salt and pepper. Set aside.

To make stacker: begin with tomato slice, top with cheese, and sprinkle with basil. Repeat.

Drizzle dressing over stackers, then top with cucumber slice, onion ring, and remaining tomato slice. Serve.

1 serving

TASTY TEN-MINUTE CHICKEN

1 tablespoon olive oil
1 boneless skinless chicken breast, cubed
Juice from 1 lemon
½ medium onion, chopped
2 cloves garlic, minced
2 plum tomatoes, chopped
2 tablespoons fresh basil
¼ teaspoon oregano
Salt and pepper to taste

In large saucepan, heat oil over medium heat and add chicken. Brown on all sides. Drizzle lemon juice over chicken and cook for 2 more minutes. Add onion and garlic, stirring until tender. Add tomatoes, basil, and oregano. Reduce heat and cook for 7 or 8 minutes, or until tomatoes are heated through.

Season with salt and pepper and serve.

1 serving

TASTY TURKEY CUTLETS

Two 3- to 4-ounce turkey breasts
1 tablespoon lemon juice
½ tablespoon olive oil
1 clove garlic, minced
¼ teaspoon dried oregano
Salt and pepper to taste

Preheat broiler.

Place turkey breasts in shallow pan.

In a small bowl, combine remaining ingredients and mix well. Pour mixture over turkey and marinate in refrigerator for 15 to 30 minutes. Broil turkey slices for 4 to 6 minutes, or until turkey is fork-tender. Serve.

2 servings

TEMPTING TURKEY HASH

1½ teaspoons olive oil
½ red or green bell pepper, chopped
½ small onion, chopped
1 medium sweet potato, diced
1 teaspoon fresh thyme
1½ cups cooked turkey, cubed
Salt and pepper to taste
3 tablespoons cream

In medium skillet, heat oil over medium heat and sauté pepper and onion approximately 2 minutes, or until softened. Add sweet potato and thyme, stirring occasionally, and cook for 10 to 12 minutes, or until potatoes are fork-tender. Add turkey, and season with salt and pepper. Slowly stir in cream and simmer for 2 to 4 minutes, or until mixture thickens. Serve.

2 servings

THREE CHEESE DIP

3 ounces cream cheese

3 ounces goat cheese

¼ cup shredded Parmesan cheese

¾ cup chopped spinach

¾ cup chopped red bell pepper

½ tablespoon chopped basil

Salt and pepper to taste

In small bowl, blend cheeses together, then add remaining ingredients. Cover and chill. Serve with cut-up vegetables or romaine lettuce leaves.

Note: This dish will keep for approximately one week in refrigerator.

Approximately 6 servings

TOMATO-TOPPED ZUCCHINI

1 tablespoon olive oil

2 small zucchini, sliced in half, lengthwise

1 plum tomato, sliced

Salt and pepper to taste

Juice of ½ lemon

6 fresh basil leaves, thinly sliced

Preheat broiler.

Lightly brush olive oil on baking sheet.

Brush zucchini halves with the remaining olive oil and broil 5 minutes. Layer tomato slices evenly over zucchini slices. Broil for another 3 to 5 minutes, or until zucchini lightly browns. Remove from oven, and season with salt and pepper. Squeeze lemon juice over each piece. Top with basil. Serve.

2 servings

TURKEY CREOLE

Two 3- to 4-ounce turkey cutlets
1 cup fresh mushrooms, washed and sliced
½ medium onion, finely chopped
3 tablespoons water
½ clove garlic, minced
½ medium green bell pepper, thinly sliced
1 cup stewed tomatoes, chopped

Preheat oven to 375 degrees. Place turkey cutlets in shallow baking dish and set aside.

In large saucepan, combine all remaining ingredients. Cook over medium heat, stirring frequently, for 10 minutes. Spread mixture evenly over turkey cutlets and bake for 20 minutes, or until turkey's juices run clear. Serve.

2 servings

TURKEY POPPERS

1 medium jalapeño pepper, seeded and halved
2 tablespoons cream cheese, separated
2 slices nitrate-free turkey bacon

Fill each jalapeño half with 1 tablespoon cream cheese. Wrap in turkey bacon.

In small pan, cook poppers over medium-high heat for 6 to 8 minutes, or until bacon is cooked. Serve.

1 serving

TWISTED CAULIFLOWER

1½ cups chicken stock
1½ teaspoons dill seed
2 bay leaves
2 cups cauliflower, cut into small chunks
1 heaping tablespoon Dijon mustard
1 teaspoon chopped dill

In large skillet, combine chicken stock, dill seed, and bay leaves. Cover and simmer. Stir in cauliflower. Cover and continue to simmer for 6 to 8 minutes, or until cauliflower reaches desired doneness.

Place cauliflower and stock in bowl, removing bay leaf. Refrigerate for 30 minutes. Drain cauliflower, retaining ⅓ cup of stock.

Combine stock, mustard, and dill. Toss cauliflower in mustard mixture and serve.

4 servings; approximately ½ cup per serving

WALDORF TURKEY SALAD

1 cup cooked turkey breast, cubed
2 celery ribs, thinly sliced
½ cup chopped Granny Smith apple
⅓ cup halved seedless grapes
¼ cup chopped walnuts
¼ cup unsweetened Greek-style yogurt
3 cups mixed greens

In large bowl, combine first 6 ingredients. Mix well. Serve over greens.

2 servings

ZUCCHINI SOUP

1 tablespoon olive oil

¼ medium sweet onion, chopped

1 clove garlic, minced

2 medium zucchini, cut into small chunks

1 cup gluten-free vegetable stock

1½ tablespoons heavy cream

In large saucepan, heat olive oil over medium heat. Add onion and garlic, and sauté until onion is translucent. Add zucchini and stock. Simmer for 6 to 9 minutes, or until zucchini is soft. Place all ingredients in blender and add cream. Puree until mixture reaches desired consistency.

2 servings

Vegetarian Recipes

If you're looking for vegetarian dishes to support your adrenals, look no further. These tasty recipes can be used to replace those with meat, poultry, or seafood as the main ingredient.

BLACK BEAN AND QUINOA SALAD

1 teaspoon olive oil

1 clove garlic, chopped

⅓ cup uncooked quinoa

¾ cup vegetable broth

1 teaspoon ground cumin

Salt and pepper to taste

Cayenne pepper (optional)

½ cup corn kernels

½ medium onion, finely chopped

1 cup canned black beans, rinsed and drained

½ cup chopped cilantro

6 scallions, chopped, using white part plus an inch of green (optional)

In large pan, heat olive oil over medium heat. Sauté garlic until lightly browned. Add quinoa and vegetable broth. Mix well. Add cumin, salt, pepper, and cayenne. Mix well. Bring mixture to a boil. Cover, reduce heat to low, and simmer 15 minutes. Stir in corn and onions. Continue to cook approximately 10 minutes, or until vegetables have softened. Mix in beans, stirring well, and heat another 2 to 3 minutes. Remove from heat and add cilantro. Garnish with scallions, if using. Serve.

4 servings

CRUNCHY TOFU STIR-FRY

½ tablespoon cornstarch
½ tablespoon chopped ginger
½ tablespoon Bragg Liquid Aminos or gluten-free soy sauce
¼ cup gluten-free chicken or turkey broth
½ tablespoon olive oil
¼ medium onion, thinly sliced
¼ medium red bell pepper, thinly sliced
½ cup broccoli
2 tablespoons cashews
½ cup firm tofu, cubed

In small bowl, combine cornstarch, ginger, soy sauce, and broth. Mix well and set aside.

In frying pan or wok, heat oil over high heat. Add onion and stir constantly for approximately 1 minute, or until onions turn translucent. Add bell pepper, broccoli, and cashews, and continue stirring until vegetables reached desired crispness. Stir in tofu and ginger mixture, and cook 4 to 6 minutes, or until sauce thickens and tofu is heated through.

1 serving

GARLIC LEMON TEMPEH

1½ tablespoons lemon juice
1 tablespoon tamari
2 cloves garlic, minced
1 teaspoon lemon zest
4 ounces tempeh, cut in bite-size cubes
2 teaspoons olive oil

In small glass bowl, combine lemon juice, tamari, garlic, and lemon zest. Mix well. Add tempeh cubes and marinate for 30 minutes on counter, or else marinate for up to 2 days in refrigerator.

In medium skillet, heat olive oil over medium heat. Add tempeh and sauté, stirring gently, for approximately 5 minutes, or until tempeh is heated through.

2 servings

ITALIAN QUICHE

1 cup chopped eggplant

½ cup chopped zucchini

½ cup chopped red bell pepper

⅓ cup chopped onion

1 clove garlic, minced

1 teaspoon olive oil, plus extra for loaf pan

4 eggs, beaten

⅓ cup heavy cream

½ cup shredded mozzarella cheese

1 teaspoon fresh oregano

½ cup chopped basil

Preheat oven to 400 degrees.

In large skillet, heat olive oil over medium heat. Sauté eggplant, zucchini, bell pepper, onion, and garlic until onion is translucent and vegetables reach desired tenderness. Remove from heat.

In medium bowl, combine eggs, cream, cheese, and spices. Stir well.

Lightly oil 7 x 11 loaf pan. Pour mixture in pan and bake for 20 minutes, or until center is set. Remove from oven and let cool 10 minutes before serving.

2 servings

MEDITERRANEAN BAKED TOFU

1 pound firm tofu, cut into thin slabs
⅓ cup olive oil
⅓ cup red-wine vinegar
2 teaspoons chopped basil
1 teaspoon chopped oregano
1 teaspoon salt
½ teaspoon freshly ground black pepper
2 plum tomatoes, cut into eight pieces
½ cup chopped onion
1 cup Kalamata olives
⅓ cup feta cheese

Drain tofu on paper towels.

In small bowl, combine olive oil, vinegar, herbs, and salt and pepper. Mix well.

In medium bowl, pour oil-and-vinegar marinade over tofu and let sit for at least 1 hour on counter, or up to overnight in refrigerator.

Preheat oven to 350 degrees.

Add tomatoes, onion, and olives to marinated tofu. Place mixture in glass casserole and bake for 20 minutes. Sprinkle feta cheese on tofu, then bake for an additional 5 to 7 minutes, or until feta cheese melts slightly.

4 servings

SAVORY QUINOA

1 cup lentils
2 cups quinoa, well rinsed
1 large onion, diced
5 cups vegetable broth
1 teaspoon dried Italian herbs
½ to 1 teaspoon sea salt

Preheat oven to 350 degrees.

Combine all ingredients in a casserole dish and bake for 45 to 60 minutes.

4 servings

TOFU AND BROCCOLI STIR-FRY

1 tablespoon olive oil
½ medium onion, finely chopped
2 cloves garlic, minced
½ block firm tofu, drained, cut into small cubes
1 cup broccoli, chopped
½-inch section of ginger, peeled and grated
Red pepper flakes (optional)
1½ tablespoons cornstarch
2 tablespoons Bragg Liquid Aminos or gluten-free soy sauce
½ cup water

In large saucepan, heat olive oil over medium-high heat. Add onions and garlic, and sauté until onions are translucent. Add tofu and broccoli and cook until broccoli reaches desired tenderness. Add ginger and red pepper flakes. Reduce heat to medium.

In small bowl, combine cornstarch, soy sauce, and water. Mix well and add to pan, stirring gently. Cook 3 to 5 minutes, or until sauce thickens.

2 servings

VEGGIE BURGER

½ medium onion, chopped

1 clove garlic, minced

1½ teaspoons olive oil

One 15-ounce can pinto beans, drained and rinsed

⅓ cup shelled sunflower seeds

1 teaspoon chopped basil

1 teaspoon salt

1½ cups cooked brown rice

In large skillet, sauté onion and garlic in ½ teaspoon olive oil until onions are translucent. Remove from pan.

In large bowl, mash pinto beans with back of fork. Add cooked onions and garlic and all remaining ingredients except olive oil and mix well. Form mixture into 4 patties.

Back in large skillet, heat remaining olive oil over medium heat. Cook patties 4 to 6 minutes per side, or until evenly browned on both sides.

4 servings

Make Your Own Yogurt

Some people enjoy making their own yogurt. The process isn't hard and you are able to produce a yogurt that has the consistency and flavor you like.

HOMEMADE YOGURT

2 cups cow or goat milk, preferably organic
½ cup plain yogurt with active cultures (see note)

In medium pan, heat milk over medium heat to approximately 200 degrees, using candy thermometer to measure temperature. Maintain temperature for 20 minutes. Remove pan from heat and cool milk to 120 degrees. (Pan can be placed in a sink filled with a few inches of cool water to help decrease the temperature.) Add plain yogurt, stirring well. Cover pan and heat at approximately 100 degrees for 4 hours, or until yogurt reaches desired consistency and flavor.

To heat yogurt, use one of the following methods:

- *Oven Method (Gas or Electric):* Heat oven to 100 degrees. Turn off oven and place pan in oven. Check temperature frequently. If oven does not maintain heat, reheat to 100 degrees. Do not leave oven on—yogurt will cook and will not culture. Yogurt is done in about 4 hours, or when thick and creamy. For extra tanginess, allow yogurt to culture for additional time.

- *Insulated Cooler Method:* Place yogurt mixture in lidded container with lid tightly sealed. Fill cooler with hot tap water, between 85 and 120 degrees, until container is half immersed. (If water cools during culturing process, add additional hot tap water to maintain temperature.) Yogurt is done about 4 hours later, when it is rich and creamy. For extra tanginess, allow yogurt to culture for additional time.

Add flavoring, stevia, or fresh fruit and enjoy!

Note: When buying yogurt with active cultures, look for *Lactobacillus bulgaricus* and *Streptococcus thermophilus*.

SOY YOGURT

4 cups soy milk
½ cup plain soy yogurt with active cultures (see note)

In large bowl or large jar, combine ingredients and mix well.

Place yogurt in a tightly sealed, lidded container and heat at 100 degrees for approximately 4 hours, or until yogurt reaches desired consistency and flavor.

To heat yogurt, use one of the following methods:

- *Oven Method (Gas or Electric):* Heat oven to 100 degrees. Transfer yogurt to oven-proof pan. Turn off oven and place pan in oven. Check temperature frequently. If oven does not maintain heat, reheat to 100 degrees. Do not leave oven on—yogurt will cook and will not culture. Yogurt is done in about 4 hours, or when thick and creamy. For extra tanginess, allow yogurt to culture for additional time.

- *Insulated Cooler Method:* Place yogurt mixture in lidded container with lid tightly sealed. Fill cooler with hot tap water, between 85 and 120 degrees, until container is half immersed. (If the water cools during the culturing process, add additional hot tap water to maintain temperature.) Yogurt is done about 4 hours later, when it is rich and creamy. For extra tanginess, allow yogurt to culture for additional time.

Add flavoring, stevia, or fresh fruit and enjoy!

Note: When buying soy yogurt with active cultures, look for *Lactobacillus bulgaricus, Streptococcus thermophilus,* or *L. Acidophilus.*

Adrenal-Friendly Treats

Now, what about dessert? Here are some sweet and satisfying treats that don't require either sugar or white flour: cakes, custards, and a type of cheesecake, as well as refreshing smoothies. There's also my favorite pizza—not a dessert, but definitely a treat. If you're looking for a healthy way to follow the 90–10 rule (see page 96), look no further: treat yourself to dessert, pizza, or a smoothie—and enjoy!

CHOCOLATE ALMOND CAKE

¼ cup (½ stick) unsalted butter, cubed, plus extra for greasing pan

4 ounces unsweetened dark chocolate, finely chopped

⅓ cup finely chopped almonds

3 eggs, separated

⅓ cup plus 1 tablespoon erythritol

½ teaspoon almond extract

Preheat oven to 375 degrees.

Lightly butter 4-inch springform pan.

Using double boiler over medium heat, melt butter and chocolate, stirring until smooth. Remove from heat and add almonds.

Mix together egg yolks and sweetener. Pour egg mixture into chocolate, stirring well. Add almond extract.

In large bowl, whip egg whites until firm peaks form. Fold egg whites into chocolate mixture, being careful not to overmix. Pour mixture into springform pan. Bake 14 to 16 minutes, or until cake is firm in center. Remove from oven and cool on cooling rack. Cool completely before cutting. Serve with fresh berries.

6 to 8 servings

EGG CUSTARD

5 large eggs
1 cup water, at room temperature
1 cup heavy cream
4 teaspoons stevia
1 teaspoon gluten-free vanilla extract
Cinnamon or nutmeg

Preheat oven to 350 degrees.

Mix all ingredients together until well blended and frothy. Pour into glass baking dish or individual oven-tempered bowls. Sprinkle with cinnamon or nutmeg. Bake for 40 to 50 minutes, or until set. Serve warm or chilled.

4 servings

LOTTA LEMON DESSERT

4 ounces cream cheese
2 tablespoons lemon juice
½ medium lemon, peeled and chopped into small chunks
½ cup stevia, or more to taste
3 cups whipped cream
¼ cup blueberries

Combine all ingredients except blueberries and blend in food processor or blender until smooth. Garnish with blueberries. Chill until firm, and serve.

2 servings

MANGO ALMOND SMOOTHIE

1 mango, cubed
1 cup ice cubes
1½ cups almond milk
1 scoop whey or soy protein powder (use the scoop that comes in the package)
Honey, stevia, erythritol, or xylitol to taste
Dash gluten-free vanilla extract

Place all ingredients in blender and process until desired consistency is reached.

For extra thickness, freeze mango cubes and process while frozen.

2 servings

MANGO SMOOTHIE

1 mango, cubed
½ cup plain Greek-style yogurt
½ cup cold water
1 scoop vanilla whey protein powder (use the scoop that comes in the package)
Stevia, erythritol, or xylitol to taste

Place all ingredients in blender and process until desired consistency is reached.

For extra thickness, freeze mango cubes and process while frozen.

2 servings

MARCELLE'S FAVORITE PIZZA

Against the Grain 12-inch gourmet frozen pizza shell
½ cup of your favorite pizza sauce
8 ounces cheese

Preheat oven to 550 degrees. Then preheat pizza stone for 30 minutes.

Fill shell with sauce and cheese, then put on preheated pizza stone. Bake 10 minutes, or until cheese is melted and golden brown. Let cool 10 minutes before serving.

4 servings; 2 slices per serving

PEANUT BUTTER BITES

1 cup creamy peanut butter
¾ cup xylitol
1 egg

Preheat oven to 350 degrees.

In medium bowl, combine all ingredients and drop dough by teaspoonfuls onto cookie sheet, 18 total. Bake 8 to 10 minutes, or until cookies set. Do not overbake! Remove immediately onto cooling rack. Cookies will be soft. Cool, then serve.

18 servings

RICOTTA DESSERT

1 cup ricotta cheese
2 tablespoons stevia, or to taste
Grated zest of 1 lemon

Whip cheese in food processor until smooth. Add sweetener and lemon zest, stirring until smooth.

Serve in individual bowls.

2 servings

SOY STRAWBERRY SMOOTHIE

½ cup vanilla soy milk
1 ounce firm silken tofu, chilled and cut into small cubes
1 cup fresh strawberries, cut into small chunks
1 scoop vanilla whey protein powder (use the scoop that comes in the package)
2 tablespoons honey, erythritol, stevia, or xylitol
¼ teaspoon gluten-free vanilla extract

Place all ingredients in blender and process until desired consistency is reached.

For added texture, freeze strawberries, and process while still frozen. Serve.

2 servings

Your Adrenal-Friendly Pantry

It's much easier sticking to an adrenal-friendly diet if you keep your kitchen well stocked with healthy foods that support your adrenals, blood sugar, and overall health and well-being. Here are some suggestions for foods to keep on hand:

- Lots of your favorite fresh or frozen vegetables—organic, if possible! As we saw on page 94, it's more important to buy organic for some foods than for others, so if you like, focus your organic purchases based on the lists on pages 94–95. You'll find it easier and more convenient to eat healthy if you keep your favorite fresh fruits and veggies washed and cut in the refrigerator for easy use. The menu plans rely more heavily on lower glycemic fruits and veggies, such as those listed below.

Fruits		
Apples	Honeydew	Plums
Blueberries	Peaches	Raspberries
Cantaloupe	Pears	Strawberries
Vegetables		
Artichokes	Cauliflower	Radishes
Asparagus	Celery	Sauerkraut
Bell peppers	Cucumbers	Spinach
Broccoli	Green beans	Squash
Brussels sprouts	Lettuce	
Cabbage	Onions	

FREEZE YOUR WAY TO ADRENAL HEALTH

Berries can be individually frozen on a cookie sheet and then transferred to freezer-friendly containers and kept for up to 12 months. Freezing the berries this way allows you to vacuum-seal whole berries and prevents clumping.

- Extra-virgin olive oil—organic if possible

- An assortment of gluten-free bread products, including crackers, rolls, and the like. See Resources for some good brands.

- A plentiful assortment of fresh or dried organic herbs

- Salt and black pepper. The best salt to use is Celtic salt, which has all the trace minerals in it, but sea salt and kosher salt are also fine.

- Lemons for zesting and juicing. Leave a few out in a bowl on your counter to use when you need fresh lemon juice. Keeping the fruit at room temperature allows the membranes to soften so juicing will be easier.

- A high-quality whey, rice, or soy protein powder for smoothies

- Filtered spring or sparkling water

- Your favorite sugar substitute—erythritol, stevia, or xylitol

- Eggs—organic if possible

- Cashews, almonds, pecans, macadamia nuts, walnuts (raw, unsalted)

- Cashew butter or almond butter

- Cheese—your favorite types, such as cheddar, ricotta, or goat cheese. Be aware that goat cheese comes in so many different varieties these days that if you don't like one, you'll surely find a type that tastes yummy.

- Brown rice

- Herbal, naturally decaffeinated teas

Shopping Lists

Concerned about how to keep an adrenal-friendly fridge and pantry? Here are the shopping lists you'll need to prepare for your 30-day adrenal-friendly eating plan:

SHOPPING LIST – Week 1		
Fruits		
Apples: Granny Smith, other	Berries: strawberries, other	Limes
Avocados	Lemons	
Vegetables		
Asparagus	Garlic	Shallots
Bell peppers: green and red	Hot peppers: jalapeño	Spinach
Broccoli	Kale	Sweet potatoes
Cucumbers	Romaine lettuce	Vegetables for dipping and salads
Escarole	Salad greens	Zucchini
Herbs/Spices		
Basil	Marjoram	Parsley
Cilantro	Mint	Thyme
Dill	Mustard	
Ginger	Oregano	
Staples		
Almond butter	Cashew butter	Lentils
Artichoke hearts	Cashews	Olive oil
Balsamic vinegar	Crackers, gluten-free	Onions
Broth: chicken or vegetable	Green chilies	Pecans
Brown rice	Hummus	Soy sauce, gluten-free
Cajun seasoning	Kalamata olives	
Dairy, Poultry, Seafood, Meats		
Butter, unsalted	Goat cheese	Shrimp
Chicken	Lamb chops	Sour cream
Cream	Parmesan cheese	Swiss cheese
Cream cheese	Pork	Turkey
Eggs	Ricotta cheese	Yogurt, Greek-style
Feta cheese	Salmon	

SHOPPING LIST – Week 2

Fruits

Apples	Grapes	Oranges
Avocados	Lemons	Other favorite fruits
Berries: raspberries, other	Melons	

Vegetables

Bell peppers: green and red	Garlic	Salad greens
Broccoli	Hot peppers: jalapeño	Spinach
Brussels sprouts	Jícama	Sweet potatoes
Celery	Mushrooms	Vegetables for dipping and salads
Cucumbers	Onions: green and red	
Escarole	Romaine lettuce	

Herbs/Spices

Basil	Marjoram	Thyme
Dill	Parsley	

Staples

Almond butter	Kalamata olives	Stewed tomatoes
Artichoke hearts	Lemon juice	Sugar substitute
Bread crumbs, gluten-free	Mayonnaise	Vanilla extract, gluten-free
Broth: chicken or vegetable	Olive oil	Walnuts
Brown rice	Pecans	Water chestnuts
Capers	Red wine vinegar	Worcestershire sauce
Cashew butter	Rolls, gluten-free	
Hummus	Soy sauce, gluten-free	

Dairy, Poultry, Seafood, Meats

Butter, unsalted	Feta cheese	Ricotta cheese
Cheddar cheese	Goat cheese	Shrimp
Chicken	Haddock	Steak

SHOPPING LIST – Week 2		
Cream	Lamb chops	Turkey
Cream cheese	Lox	Turkey bacon, nitrate-free
Eggs	Parmesan cheese	Yogurt, Greek-Style

SHOPPING LIST – Week 3		
Fruits		
Apples	Grapes	Melons
Avocados	Lemons	Tomatoes
Berries: raspberries, strawberries	Limes	
Vegetables		
Asparagus	Escarole	Salad greens
Bell peppers: green and red	Garlic	Spinach
Broccoli	Hot peppers: jalapeño	Sweet potatoes
Brussels sprouts	Kale	Vegetables for dipping and salads
Cauliflower	Mushrooms	Zucchini
Celery	Onions: green, red, and Vidalia	
Cucumbers	Romaine lettuce	
Herbs/Spices		
Basil	Ginger	Paprika
Bay leaves	Marjoram	Parsley
Cilantro	Mustard	Red pepper flakes
Curry powder	Old Bay seasoning	Thyme
Dill	Oregano	
Staples		
Almond butter	Grains: millet, quinoa	Protein powder: whey or soy
Artichoke hearts	Green chilies	Rice: brown and white
Balsamic vinegar	Hot sauce	Rolls, gluten-free

SHOPPING LIST – Week 3

Bread, gluten-free	Hummus	Soy sauce, gluten-free
Broth: chicken or vegetable	Kalamata olives	Stewed tomatoes
Capers (optional)	Lemon juice	Walnuts
Cashew butter	Olive oil	Water chestnuts
Cornstarch	Onions	White wine
Crackers, gluten-free	Pecans	Worcestershire sauce

Dairy, Poultry, Seafood, Meats

Chicken	Haddock	Sour cream
Crabmeat	Lamb chops	Steak
Cream	Mozzarella cheese	Swiss cheese
Cream cheese	Parmesan cheese	Turkey
Eggs	Ricotta cheese	Turkey bacon, nitrate-free
Feta cheese	Salmon: fresh and cured (lox)	Yogurt, Greek-style
Goat cheese	Shrimp	

SHOPPING LIST – Week 4

Fruits

Apples: Granny Smith, other	Grapes	Melons
Avocados	Lemons	Tomatoes and plum tomatoes
Berries: strawberries, other	Limes	

Vegetables

Asparagus	Garlic	Salad greens
Bell peppers: green and red	Hot peppers: jalapeño	Spinach
Broccoli	Kale	Sweet potatoes
Celery	Onions: green, shallot, and Vidalia	Vegetables for dipping and salad
Cucumber	Pea pods	
Escarole	Romaine lettuce	

SHOPPING LIST – Week 4

Herbs/Spices

Basil	Ginger	Paprika
Bay leaves	Marjoram	Parsley
Cilantro	Mustard	Thyme
Dill	Nutmeg	

Staples

Almond butter	Crackers, gluten-free	Protein powder: whey or soy
Artichoke hearts	Grains: millet, quinoa	Rice, brown
Balsamic vinegar	Green chilies	Rolls, gluten-free
Bread, gluten-free	Hot sauce	Soy sauce, gluten-free
Broth: chicken or vegetable	Hummus	Stewed tomatoes
Capers (optional)	Kalamata olives	Walnuts
Cashew butter	Olive oil	Water chestnuts
Cornstarch	Onions	White wine

Dairy, Poultry, Seafood, Meats

Butter, unsalted	Goat cheese	Sour cream
Cheese, your favorite	Haddock	Steak
Chicken	Lamb chops	Swiss cheese
Crabmeat	Mozzarella cheese	Turkey
Cream	Parmesan cheese	Turkey bacon, nitrate-free
Cream cheese	Ricotta cheese	Yogurt, Greek-style
Eggs	Salmon: fresh and cured (lox)	
Feta cheese	Shrimp	

Making Sure Your Diet Is Effective

Nothing is more discouraging than being disciplined about your eating plan and not losing the weight you'd like—only because you aren't appropriately supporting your adrenal-friendly food choices with healthy lifestyle and exercise choices. To make sure you're doing everything you can to support your adrenals and achieve or maintain your ideal weight, turn to Chapter 7.

EXERCISE AND LIFESTYLE

"I'm a real gym rat," Madison told me as soon as she sat down for our first appointment. "I take a spinning class three times a week, step aerobics the other two days, and on the weekend, I work out on the treadmill. I'm *really* good about never missing a day. So why am I gaining weight? And why do I feel so tired all the time? I feel like my body is just turning against me."

Madison was a 32-year-old corporate human resources manager, a demanding position that involved constant negotiations between employees and different levels of management. She had just started a relationship with a man at work, and while their office romance wasn't exactly forbidden, they were trying to be discreet about it. Madison was eager to have children, so she was very much hoping this guy was "the one." When I asked her about the important people in her life, she told me that her best friend, whom she'd known since college, had recently been diagnosed with cancer.

Madison was a Racehorse: someone whose cortisol and DHEA levels stayed high throughout the day. As a result, her seemingly abundant energy masked a serious problem with adrenal dysfunction, which was exacerbated by a number of stressors in her life: her work, her relationship, and her seriously ill best friend. Although exercise can often be a wonderful stress release, in some circumstances it can instead add to our stress and overwork our adrenals. This was Madison's situation, as I tried to explain to her.

At first, Madison just stared at me in disbelief. "You mean I have to stop going to the gym?" she kept repeating. "But that's the only thing that's keeping me sane!"

I tried to explain to Madison that in her case, too much vigorous exercise was actually serving to throw her body, mind, and spirit out of balance. If exercise makes you more tired—if you are not energized by it—then it is not helpful. Unlike Workhorses and Flatliners, Racehorses like Madison can still engage in *some* vigorous exercise. But in my opinion, she was failing to listen to her body and was therefore pushing herself far too hard.

I began to explain to her the framework I've shared throughout this book: that we need to let our soothing parasympathetic nervous system take over occasionally, that too much stress cues our body to go into "emergency" mode. But Madison kept shaking her head. "You're telling me that if I exercise too much, I'll get fat," she kept repeating. "But if I *don't* exercise, I'll get even fatter. What am I supposed to do?"

The Benefits of Gentle Exercise

Counterintuitive though it may seem, excess exercise can actually cause you to retain weight. Just as cutting too many calories can cause your body to cry, "Famine!" over-exercise can make your body think, "Emergency!" *You* know you're not taking a dangerous trek through a hostile environment, but your body behaves as though you are, holding on to every ounce of body fat for dear life—literally.

That is not to say *don't* exercise, or even that you won't someday be able to engage in vigorous activity. Exercise has so many benefits, I want to encourage you to find a type of exercise you enjoy, so you can reap the benefits, too. Getting appropriate regular exercise will:

- Help you sleep

- Boost your immune system

- Reduce your stress

- Improve your mood

- Regulate your blood pressure

- Decrease your risk of heart disease, diabetes, and osteoporosis

- Help you to live longer

- Improve your muscle tone

- Help maintain your health as you age

Yes, exercise is good for you. Your body, after all, was designed to move. So please don't deprive yourself of the joys of exercise! However, if you are experiencing adrenal dysfunction, you need to gear your level of activity accordingly. Once your adrenals are healed and your HPA axis is back in balance, you can consider a more vigorous routine.

For Madison, the idea of treating her body gently sounded "soft" and "undisciplined." As we talked further, I could hear how the idea of gaining even a single pound made her anxious and how much she regarded her body as a treacherous enemy rather than a beloved friend.

As I got to know Madison better, I came to learn that her mother, too, had been obsessed with diet, exercise, and weight. Madison's father had had a gambling problem and was frequently out of town on mysterious trips. Madison had absorbed her mother's belief that much of his reason for going was because Madison's mother had gained weight since having children, causing her to become less attractive. When Madison's father was gone, her mother "fell apart completely," in Madison's words, "barely able to get dinner on the table or to get us off to school in the morning." As the oldest child, Madison had become a kind of surrogate mother to her younger brother and sister. Her way of exerting control over her world, I began to realize, was through strictly controlling and monitoring every bite of food she put into her mouth. Even so, she relied upon exercise to remain at her ideal weight.

As a result, Madison was devastated to realize that the carefully controlled regimen she had created for herself was no longer working. Nor was her attempt to control her body helping her to cope with her relationship anxieties, her fears of not finding the right guy in time to have children, or the potential loss of her best friend. In effect, her body was screaming at her, "You have to find another way!"

Getting to the Heart of the Matter

As I was preparing this book, I seemed to hear one news story after another about women's need to exercise intensely, vigorously, and for long periods of time. One day

I heard a national news story reporting that women need to exercise an hour a day to prevent future weight gain—not even to lose any of their current weight.

If you've heard this or similar stories, I urge you not to listen. Struggling with adrenal dysfunction means that you need to gear your exercise to an appropriate level until you are completely healed. And once you and your adrenals are completely healthy, 20 minutes a day, four or five days a week of circuit or "burst" training is really all you need. If you're "bursting"—pushing yourself to your limit alternating with cool-down periods—you frustrate your body's tendency to homeostasis, which causes your body to accommodate to any stable level of exercise. Bursting enables you to exercise for only 20 minutes and get the same results as from longer, more consistent periods of exertion.

If you are eating a healthy diet and getting 20 minutes of exercise four or five times a week, and you're still not happy with your weight, the solution is not to ramp up the exercise but to figure out why your body is holding on so intensely to every ounce of fat. If your adrenal problem is solved, perhaps you're dealing with a food allergy, inflammation, a thyroid abnormality, a hormonal or neurotransmitter imbalance, a digestive issue, or detox issues. If the suggestions in this book aren't enough to help you start making progress, take a look at *The Core Balance Diet* for additional types of dietary healing; or consult with a nutritionist, naturopath, or functional-medicine specialist to find out what your body is telling you—and what you can do to respond.

Your Adrenal Exercise Plan

Because every woman reading this book is different, I will suggest an approach to figuring out what type of exercise is right for you rather than presenting a rigid plan. Here are some guidelines, followed by a few specific suggestions. But please, above all, *listen to your body.* Let it tell you what it needs and what it wants, without pushing it too hard. Don't treat your body like a bad boyfriend who needs to be scolded and manipulated and regarded with suspicion. Treat your body with love, gentleness, and care—and if it tells you it's tired and doesn't want to be pushed, believe it! In the long run, you'll look better, feel better, and heal better.

- *For Mild Adrenal Symptoms:* Choose an aerobic workout of your choice and try it for a 20-minute session, with mild weight training twice a week. Be sure to pace yourself. If you feel invigorated after your exercise, it's probably fine. If you feel exhausted afterward or later that evening, you've probably done too much.

- *For Moderate Adrenal Symptoms:* Brisk walking, three to seven times a week, 15 to 30 minutes a day. You still want to keep your heart rate below 90 beats per minute, but a mild sense of exertion is all right.

- *For Severe Adrenal Symptoms:* Slow walking, three to seven times a week, 15 to 30 minutes a day. You don't want your heart rate to go above 90 beats per minute.

ADRENAL-FRIENDLY EXERCISE PRINCIPLES

- Notice how you feel after a session. If you feel pleasantly tired and, soon after, energized, you're doing well. You can continue at your current rate or gradually step up the pace. If you feel exhausted for a few hours afterward, you've done too much. Ease up the next day and wait a while before increasing your routine.

- Find exercise you enjoy. You can put on some of your favorite music and dance around the house, take a walk in a neighborhood or outdoor spot you appreciate, share a game or sport with people you like—anything that seems like a treat instead of a punishment.

- Work exercise into your daily schedule. You might do something as simple as parking a few extra blocks from work or taking one flight of stairs up and two flights down instead of using the elevator. Exercise is effective in segments as brief as 5 minutes each, so if you can't spare 20 minutes a day, perhaps you can manage one or two 5-minute segments.

- Give yourself permission to do less than "everything." Some people find it hard to exercise at all if they can't make the time for an entire session. When my patients give themselves permission to have a shorter walk or a briefer workout, they tend to exercise far more and to feel less pressured about it.

Bursting: Fitness in 20 Minutes a Day

If you're ready for a more intense workout, you can save time and build stamina with this approach. Science has shown that if you exercise in too regular a rhythm, your metabolism adapts and eventually the weight-loss or weight-maintenance effects level off. By contrast, varying the intensity of your exercise—using a technique known as "bursting"—keeps your metabolism turned up to its highest level.

One easy way to practice bursting is to buy a small, portable step machine known as the X-iser that varies the intensity of each step (see Resources). I have one that I love because it's easy to take with me even when I travel. You can do a 20-minute session on it, or a few 5-minute sessions, which can be a wonderful way to blow off steam and unwind. If you have a type of exercise you prefer, vary your own routine in a "bursting" pattern:

- For walking, pace yourself by city blocks or telephone poles, alternating between a brisk walk and a sprint, or between a medium walk and a "race-walk," pole by pole, or block by block.

- For a treadmill workout, try one minute at, say, four miles an hour, and then one at, say, seven miles an hour, alternating minute by minute. If that is too intense a workout for you, try alternating between three and five miles an hour or build in longer rest times.

- For a very brief bursting workout, perhaps at work, try running up one flight of stairs, then walking slowly down the stairs, then running back up. Continue for 5 minutes, 10 minutes, or any length of time you have, up to 20 minutes. Four 5-minute sessions a day may be all the exercise you need.

- Here's the routine I'm currently using, and am extremely happy with: Warm up for two to three minutes. Then exercise for 30 seconds so hard that you're short of breath, followed by 90 seconds of a relaxed pace, continuing that 30–90 ratio throughout your workout. You only need to do this for a total of 20 minutes, or about eight repetitions. After even a brief time of using this method, I could feel my metabolic pathways shifting so dramatically, it was simply incredible! When you're ready for a vigorous workout, try it yourself and see.

The Healing Powers of Sleep

As Madison and I continued to work together, we also addressed her growing "sleep debt." A true Racehorse, Madison was used to working hard and playing hard, staying up late with her boyfriend or a group of girlfriends, and then going in to work early the next day after only a few hours of sleep. I was amazed at how well she seemed to function—but her weight gain and other symptoms were eloquent testimony to her body's need for rest.

Healing adrenal dysfunction, along with the symptoms that accompany it, is virtually impossible if you're not getting adequate sleep each night. Individual needs vary, but most people need between seven and nine hours per night, though some of us can make do with six and others really need ten. If you are struggling with adrenal dysfunction, you may need more sleep during recovery than you will later on, so, as always, try to be patient and gentle with yourself as you seek to extend your hours of rest.

Like Madison, most of my patients find it difficult to make adequate time for sleep, just as they find it hard to make time for exercise, relaxation, or "me time." If that is the case with you, consider that it will be extremely difficult—perhaps even impossible—to lose unwanted weight unless you are getting sufficient sleep. Your body understands lack of sleep as another one of those emergencies that causes it to hunker down and hold on to every last calorie, just as it would if you were trekking across the tundra or fleeing through the jungle.

Lack of sleep also tends to give the amygdala primacy while slighting the cerebral cortex. When you're tired, your intense, impulsive emotional brain is likely to perceive more emergencies, with less of a chance for your calm rational brain to weigh in. As a result, your amygdala may be signaling your HPA axis to send out stress hormones far more often, with no cerebral cortex activity to counter that message and invoke your soothing parasympathetic nervous system. You really *do* have a hard time thinking clearly and keeping things in perspective when you're tired—that's not a lack of discipline or willpower, but a function of how our brains are wired—and that difficulty translates into greater strain on the adrenals and more stress hormones in your system.

What if you are making time for sleep but restful sleep doesn't come, either because you can't fall asleep or because you can't remain so? In that case, it may be time to consider your *sleep hygiene*. Here are some suggestions:

- *Eat a bedtime snack.* To keep your blood sugar from falling too low during the night, have a bite to eat about an hour before bedtime, including some protein and perhaps a small amount of complex carbohydrates. As we saw in Chapter 5, these types of foods take longer to digest, helping to keep your blood sugar at a nice even level. Avoid starchy, white-flour, and sugary foods, as these will send your blood sugar spiking and then, a few hours later, crashing, which can interfere with your sleep. Some fruit is okay, if you have some protein with it, but avoid the overly sweet fruits, such as dates, figs, grapes, and bananas, choosing instead citrus, berries, apples, or pears.

- *Block out noise and light.* Make sure you're sleeping in a comfortable, quiet, and dark place. If noise interferes with your sleep, consider earplugs or a bedside "noise machine" of soothing sounds—anything from the sound of falling rain to indeterminate white noise—to cover surrounding noise. (See Resources for some suggestions.) If you live near streetlights, buy blackout curtains to shut out all nighttime light as well as the early-morning dawn. Cue your body to recognize nighttime and darkness as the time for rest.

- *Protect your sleep environment.* As you prepare for bed and fall asleep, you will find it more relaxing if you have nothing to look at but pleasant, soothing sights. Keep work-related materials or anything that demands an effort in another room, or at the very least, out of sight. It's hard to enjoy soothing, restful sleep if the last thing you see before closing your eyes is an unfinished, overdue report or a pile of unpaid bills. Keep your sleep area free of clutter and make your bedroom a true place of rest—yummy colors, no computer, nothing too stimulating—so that you genuinely feel able to release and relax when you slip into bed. You also want your sleep environment to really symbolize you, so that you feel at peace the moment you enter.

- *Avoid electronics before bedtime.* Stay away from computers, televisions, cell-phone screens, and other electronic visuals at least an hour before you plan to sleep. The flickering light behind the screen stimulates your brain to stay awake. If you're used to falling asleep in front of the TV, be aware that the flickering light is perceived through your lids and interferes with the depth and restfulness of your sleep. And of course, working on the computer or texting on your cell phone can be stimulating if not anxiety-provoking as well.

- *Develop a nighttime routine.* Especially if you have trouble falling asleep, you may find it helpful to do the same thing in the same sequence every night. This will ease your sympathetic nervous system while cuing your parasympathetic nervous system to take over. Some people can shift gears quickly and need only a 10- or 15-minute routine; others need to start winding down at least an hour before bed. Listen to your body and create the routine that is right for you. Choose soothing, calming activities—for some people, even reading is too stimulating.

- *Keep bed for sleeping (or sex!).* If you have trouble falling asleep or staying asleep, work on associating bed with sleep and rest. If you wake up in the night and can't fall back asleep within about 10 minutes or so, get up and read or do something soothing—but do it out of bed. Only return to bed when you think you might be able to sleep.

- *Think about something else.* Studies have shown that when people try to fall asleep, they have difficulty doing so. If they are able to focus on something else—say, a detailed memory of a beautiful, relaxing place, or an intricate fantasy of a happy event—their natural tiredness often takes over. If you lie in bed trying to solve the problems of your day or trying to force yourself to sleep, you'll likely be awake for hours. Either get out of bed to take action on your problems—perhaps making a list or actually completing a task—or direct your mind to a fantasy or memory that makes you feel good. A soothing visualization can be helpful as well. (See Resources for some supportive websites and visualization aids.) You may also find cognitive behavioral therapy helpful for sleep problems. (For more information, see www.cbtforinsomnia.com.)

The Herbal Pharmacy: Sleep Issues

As we have seen, insufficient sleep can play havoc with your adrenals, as well as make it extremely difficult to lose weight. So good, deep regular sleep is crucial for your overall well-being, including your adrenal health.

I don't usually recommend prescription sleep aids for my patients, as they may become habit-forming. Neither prescription nor over-the-counter sleep aids will give you the same kind of deep restful sleep that you can get on your own. I'd rather see my patients—and you—learn to find ways to de-stress and to cue the parasympathetic nervous system to take over, though I will prescribe sleep aids when needed.

Still, while you are trying to shift into a more adrenal-friendly lifestyle, you may need some additional help, so here are some herbal remedies you might use in the interim. None are habit-forming, though some have side effects that might be problematic for people with certain conditions. Try them in the following order:

- *Phosphorylated serine.* This is a brain nutrient that helps to balance the HPA axis, especially while you sleep. I find this nutrient particularly helpful, as it quiets the chatter and decreases adrenal activity, allowing you to sleep soundly. It's also very effective for bringing down high cortisol levels. The phosphorylated serine combination that I use consists of calcium (105 mg), magnesium (105 mg), phosphorus (355 mg), and l-serine (105 mg). When you find a formulation similar to this (see Resources for some companies that make useful products), take two capsules at night 30 to 60 minutes before bed.

- *Melatonin.* If the phosphorylated serine doesn't make you sleepy, then add 1 mg to 3 mg of melatonin—again, taken at night before bed. As your body prepares to sleep, melatonin levels naturally rise, cued by darkness as well as by your circadian rhythms. With age, melatonin levels often decrease, making it more difficult to sleep. If you're traveling, supplementing with melatonin can be an excellent way to reset your circadian clock and avoid jet lag: take some as your overnight flight begins or when it's nighttime in your new destination. At home, a melatonin supplement might give your body that extra sleep-inducing boost you need.

- *Calcium and magnesium.* I often suggest this combination to patients with restless leg syndrome. Taking 1,200 mg of calcium and 600 mg of magnesium may bring you some relief from the restless legs. In my experience, this syndrome often indicates either an iron deficiency or small-bowel overgrowth of bacteria. Talk to your practitioner about these possibilities.

- *5-HTP.* This extraordinary chemical is a precursor of serotonin, the biochemical that prevents depression, boosts self-esteem and optimism, and regulates sleep cycles, among other functions. If you're struggling with insomnia and/or depression, try also taking 50 mg to 150 mg of 5-HTP each day—about an hour before bedtime if you're using it as a sleep aid. Be mindful that sometimes, if you're struggling with anxiety, this supplement may make the anxiety worse.

You can combine any of the supplements I've just listed. But if they're not working as you would like, stop taking all of them and try the following supplements: first GABA, then, if that doesn't work, the combination product I suggest below. Don't combine the supplements with each other or with any others, except possibly calcium and magnesium for restless leg syndrome:

- *GABA.* GABA is short for *gamma-aminobutyric acid,* a biochemical that the body uses to induce sleep and to calm the system. 5-H GABA is precursor to GABA that is actually a more usable form that can be taken in smaller doses. A 100 mg dose of 5-H GABA taken about 30 minutes before bed can be very effective, but *avoid it if you have low blood pressure.* If you don't see results in two weeks, you can increase the dose to 200 mg. If neither dose of 5-H GABA works, try 500 mg of the straight GABA. If after two weeks you don't see results, you can increase to 1,000 mg. Be aware that if you take too much of any form of GABA, you may find yourself feeling agitated or aggressive, so start with the smallest dose and increase gradually as needed. Be prepared to cut back if you can't tolerate the side effects.

- *Combination product.* Phenylbutyric acid is a derivative of GABA, while taurine helps increase GABA activity. One compound I sometimes recommend includes a proprietary product known as Thera Mix, a combination of taurine and 4-amino-3-phenylbutyric acid, as well as 2 mg of vitamin B_6. A number of companies also offer natural sleep aids. For more information, check out the Resources.

The Herbal Pharmacy: Anxiety

Bouts of panic or anxiety also tend to strain the adrenals, so let me suggest some supplements that can be helpful in calming and soothing your mind and emotions. As we've seen, GABA can ease sleep problems and relieve anxiety. Try taking a daily dose of 100 mg of 5-H GABA along with a small piece of fruit and some protein. If this is not enough to calm you down, increase your dosage to 200 mg. Another option is to use plain GABA—between 500 mg and 750 mg per day. Again, make sure you take it with fruit and protein.

If neither version of GABA works for you, look for a compound that includes such ingredients as:

- Rehmannia root (*Rehmannia glutinosa*)

- Schisandra fruit (*Schisandra chinensis*)

- Jujube fruit (*Zizyphus spinosa*)

- Dong Quai root (*Angelica sinensis*)

- Chinese asparagus root (*Asparagus cochinchinensis*)

- Ophiopogon root (*Ophiopogon japonicus*)

- Scrophularia root (*Scrophularia ningpoensis*)

- Asian ginseng root (*Panax ginseng*)

- Chinese salvia root (*Salvia miltiorrhiza*)

- Poria fungus (*Wolfiporia cocos*)

- Polygala root (*Polygala tenuifolia*)

- Platycodon root (*Platycodon grandiflorum*)

Alternatively, look for a product that contains:

- Vitamin B_6, 25 mg

- Magnesium, 200 mg

- Taurine, 1,000 mg

- N-acetylcysteine, 600 mg

- Green tea leaf extract, decaffeinated, 300 mg

- Valerian tea is also very helpful for anxiety, as is valerian in homeopathic drops.

For all supplements, use with care and be ready to seek help from a health-care practitioner if you suffer from any side effects, especially unusual anxiety, depression, or other mental or emotional effects.

Body Work

As Madison struggled to cut back on her exercise and give her body some much-needed rest, she looked for less strenuous replacements. I suggested that she consider one or more of the following types of body work, some more active than others, to develop a gentler, more loving relationship with her body. Whether you exercise a lot, a little, or not at all, I invite you, too, to explore your body through one or more of these modalities. Experiment to see which appeals to you, or vary your choices if that feels like more of a treat.

- *Massage.* There are so many different types of massage; I could take up an entire book describing them all! To find a person or spa that is right for you, ask your friends if they have someone to recommend; check out ads at a local health-food store, dance studio, yoga studio, or gym; or look online to see whose listing catches your fancy. You can also buy one of several good books on "do-it-yourself" massage and ask a romantic partner or a friend to do "massage exchanges" with you.

- *Acupuncture and acupressure.* Acupuncture is a healing technique practiced for millennia in traditional Chinese medicine. It is based on stimulating the body's energy pathways with tiny hair-thin needles. The needles don't hurt—and they do have a remarkably restorative effect. Acupressure is a variation that involves pressure, rather than needles, at key points. Check ads or ask around at health-food stores, yoga studios, or look online for an accredited practitioner in your community.

- *Yoga.* As with massage, there are many different styles of yoga. An ancient Indian system of connecting the body to its energy sources, yoga originated as a spiritual as well as a physical discipline, but in the United States you can find everything from "power yoga"—an especially vigorous workout—to restorative yoga, a series of poses that are meant to be simple yet powerful in their ability to restore your energy, as the name suggests. If you are suffering from moderate or severe adrenal dysfunction, I recommend that you begin with restorative yoga as a profound yet gentle way to reconnect with your body—and to invite your parasympathetic nervous system to take over.

- *Tai chi.* Tai chi is another ancient form of exercise practiced in Asia that involves moving very slowly from pose to pose in a kind of moving meditation. Some forms of tai chi are vigorous and demanding, while others are gentler. For those of us who like to move fast, tai chi can be an excellent way to encourage ourselves to slow down.

- *Qigong.* Pronounced "chi gung," qigong is another ancient Chinese martial art with healing properties. Qigong relies on a system of breathing to mobilize the energy in body and spirit, along with other types of mental and physical training. Qigong practitioners claim that the practice brings relaxation, an increased sense of spiritual satisfaction, and numerous benefits to physical health and well-being.

Do Your Heart Math

One device that I have personally found very helpful is the emWave, manufactured by HeartMath. The emWave machine gives you immediate feedback on your stress levels by performing *heart rate variability analysis* (HRV)—that is, by measuring the subtle changes in your heart rhythms. You put your finger in the device to get a reading on your heart rhythm, since the more stressed you are, the more variable your rhythm is likely to be. Because you're getting instant feedback, you can learn to put yourself into a more relaxed state in which your heart rate becomes more even and balanced. For more information, see the Resources.

Environmental Stress

So far, we've been talking about the stresses of our daily life. But there's another type of stress that can affect our adrenal balance, which is *environmental stress.* More and more of the women I treat seem to be having difficulties with a wide range of environmental stressors, from household cleaning products to the metals in their dental work.

It's uncomfortable to realize that our own homes may be minefields of potentially toxic products. Cosmetics, shampoo, water bottles, microwaves, and the linings in cans of foods contain chemicals that put a low-grade strain on all of us and may have more severe effects on women with weakened immune systems, greater sensitivities, or unbalanced adrenal systems. Likewise, power lines, computers, cell phones, televisions, and other electronic devices create electromagnetic fields to which some people are sensitive.

Heavy metals have become another source of concern for many of my patients. In addition to the potential dangers of heavy-metal contamination in fish, groundwater, and the environment, many of us face possible problems from heavy metals in our mouths, where they are often used for dental amalgams, fillings, and other dental work.

Our own drinking water may pose problems, too. I was shocked to learn recently that because of the high use of prescription medications among the population as a whole, many of us are drinking from water supplies with a relatively high concentration of antibiotics, hormones, and antidepressants. Other medical waste, including leftover prescription drugs and even chemotherapy products used at home, is sometimes simply flushed down the toilet, where again, it can get into our drinking water.

As we saw in Chapter 5, food may also be a source of toxins. Additives and preservatives put a strain on the liver, which filters out bodily toxins. These days, a surprisingly high percentage of food is irradiated and/or genetically modified. Although no large long-term studies have yet been done on these relatively recent developments, some evidence indicates that many people—especially those with allergies or other autoimmune conditions—react badly to the artificially created proteins in genetically modified foods, with potentially stressful results.

Each of us responds differently, of course. But if you're suffering from adrenal dysfunction, your response to environmental toxins may be a factor, either creating or aggravating your condition through their burden on your adrenal glands.

It's not as though any of us could escape the chemical assault. According to a shocking report known as the BodyBurden study, some 287 industrial chemicals and pollutants can be found in the cord blood of the average newborn. Likewise, a Maine study called the Body of Evidence analyzed the blood and hair of several Maine residents, including some legislators—and not one person had normal values. As a longtime resident of Maine, I was struck by a report by the state fish and wildlife departments warning women who were pregnant or planning to become so to eat local fish only once a month—because of the toxic chemicals they contain. In addition, CNN recently reported that because so many meats are riddled with pesticides, organic meats may be a safer choice.

Our own homes may be toxic minefields because of the many seemingly innocent products they contain. To take just one example, Bisphenol A (BPA) is used to make polycarbonate plastic and epoxy resins, which in turn are used in numerous products, including baby bottles, water bottles, metal can liners, medical and dental devices, eyeglass lenses, dental fillings, sports equipment, CDs and DVDs, and household electronics. Bisphenol A is a known endocrine disruptor whose estrogenic effects can mimic the body's own hormones and cause negative health effects. Concern over BPA and human consumption was raised both by The Endocrine Society in 2009 and the U.S. Food and Drug Administration in 2010. (For more information, see www.nih.gov and www.ewg.org.)

Again, I'm not trying to scare you. But I am hoping that with this new understanding, you can take new actions. If you think that you may be suffering from environmental sensitivities, I urge you to see a specialist in functional medicine or a naturopath (someone who uses herbal and other natural supplements to restore the body's balance). You can also read more about how hidden toxins may be affecting you and your family. (For help with all of these issues, see Resources.) Meanwhile, give some thought to eliminating as many environmental toxins as you can from your diet and your home. Your adrenal glands will be grateful—and your health may improve as a result!

Economic Stress and the 24-Hour Workday

When my patient Sofia came to see me, she looked exhausted. She'd been tested for adrenal dysfunction at her last visit and now she was here to get the results. I started explaining to her that she did indeed have adrenal dysfunction and that she might need to build in some time each day for de-stressing, and she just shook her head and looked at me.

"I'm already working two jobs because the economy is so bad," she finally said. "We have a sitter sometimes, but not always—we just can't always afford it. So Hector has to pick up the kids from school, or I do—and he's only getting day work now, so sometimes he can, but when he has a job, then it's up to me—and when it was just *one* job I could manage, but now that I have two!"

She barely paused for breath before she began again. "Every week, I think I'm going to go crazy with the bills piling up—I try to pay a little each week, but I can't always manage that. Last week, my daughter was going to a birthday party and I just didn't have the heart to tell her she couldn't get her friend a present, but we really couldn't afford it."

She took another breath and forced herself to stop. "Relaxing, that sounds good," she said with an attempt at a wry smile. "But how am I supposed to manage it?"

GOING GREEN AT HOME

If you think you're struggling with environmental sensitivities—or if you just want to live in a cleaner, safer environment, try these basic steps for a greener life at home:

- Don't microwave food in plastic containers—use glass or ceramic ones instead.

- Don't store foods in plastic containers—use covered glass or ceramic dishes or bowls.

- Use "green" cleaning products instead of the kind that contain toxic chemicals. (See Resources for some suggestions.)

- Try substituting small fish (sardines, trout, whiting) for large ones (tuna, swordfish, salmon) to avoid the mercury that tends to be found in the larger fish.

- Avoid genetically modified and irradiated foods. (For more information about these types of foods, see Resources.)

- See a biological dentist for an evaluation of your mercury fillings and/or have a heavy-metal evaluation done.

- Eat organic as much as possible. Clean out your pantry and get rid of processed and additive-laden foods.

- If possible, use additive-free cosmetics and skin-care products. (See Resources.)

I wish I could say that Sofia was the only patient to come to me with this kind of story. Unfortunately, more and more of my patients have to balance two jobs and have to work twice as hard at their jobs as they did before, both to compensate for people who have been laid off and to make sure that they won't be the next ones to go. These are very real problems, as is the stress they generate. Once you lose the locus of control for your own and your family's life, your stress level skyrockets.

In fact, statistics show that the effects of stress are more harmful when we feel a lack of control over our lives—and being uncertain of our ability to support ourselves is one very significant way we feel out of control. Poverty also tends to exacerbate stress because of the constant economic, social, and personal challenges, such as the ones Sofia described, and because in the United States, it often tends to isolate us and cut us off from social supports. In other countries with different attitudes about money, class, and wealth, poverty feels like more of a communal experience—challenging on a daily basis, but not creating the sense of isolation, helplessness, and failure with which so many of my patients struggle.

Now I needed to speak to Sofia's current situation, suggesting ways she might heal her adrenals without ignoring the very real economic challenges she was facing.

"I'm so sorry," I told Sofia. "I can only imagine how hard your situation is right now. I suggest to some of my patients that they need to cut back on some of their work and take more time for *them*. But I can see that right now, you need every hour of work you can get. I'll suggest an adrenal-friendly diet and some nutritional supplements that will definitely help restore your energy.

"But let's also try to make *some* time for you in there. I can suggest simple things to do during the day, even while you're working. For example, massaging your earlobes and the top part of your temple, even a few times a day, will help ease your stress. I can also show you some breathing exercises that you can do in a minute or two. Finding just two or three times a day to do them will make a big difference. Meditation can also help, even if only two minutes at a time, twice a day. If we work together, we can absolutely find a way to give you some downtime, so your system can rebalance and heal."

Sofia agreed to give my suggestions a try. When I thought about her situation, I was struck by the number of women I know who are constantly working—or feel that they *should* be. In addition to the economic pressures that Sofia was feeling, there are all the women who are still hearing the echoes of Mom or Dad telling them, "You're just not good enough," and driving themselves mercilessly in an effort to prove their parents wrong. For many of us, perfectionism, the need to control, or the feeling that we've never quite done enough are the sad legacy of parents who seemed frequently dissatisfied with us—even though our parents were themselves responding to *their* parents, doing the best they could with what they were given. Understand that our parents were "guilty, but not to blame," as were their parents. The legacy goes on for generations—until we stop it.

Our culture, too, puts a lot of pressure on us to be constantly working. If you go to a party in the United States, the first thing most people will ask you is, "What do you do?" In Europe, where the culture is less work-obsessed, that's actually considered an offensive question, as I once learned to my embarrassment. A fellow guest at a party I once attended in Amsterdam actually took me aside and scolded me for asking another guest about his occupation. "Don't you know that there is so much more to a person than just his job?" he asked me. "Why are you Americans so concerned with work all the time? You never get to know who the person *is,* just what they do." While I think a person's job can be an important part of his or her identity, I saw my host's point. When you define yourself by your job, it's hard to find the courage to stop working—even though most of us, in my professional opinion, are working far too hard!

Remember, the human body was never designed for constant unremitting stress. It was meant to exert itself, rise to the occasion, and then have a chance to relax. In "the old days," when people lived by candlelight and depended upon their own biological clocks, we got up with the sun, worked hard, and then spent the evening preparing for sleep.

I'm not suggesting a return to those pre-electric times, but I do think a compromise is in order. I was so amazed, whenever our family lost power for a night or two, at how much more fun we had together. We lit candles, played games, talked, and shared our lives in a way that just doesn't happen now that we have computers, TVs, and telephones to occupy our every minute. I wouldn't want to be without power for *too* long—but once in a while might not be so bad.

Consider an Electronic Sabbath

One way to cue your parasympathetic nervous system to take over—and perhaps also to reconnect with your partner and family—is to give yourself an *electronic Sabbath:* all or part of your weekend with no electronic media. If that seems too challenging, perhaps cut out the work-related media. Get separate e-mails for personal and work use, and check only your personal account.

I also know people who have instituted "Facebook Sabbaths," when they avoid social networking for one evening a week or for the weekend, or "Browser Sabbaths," when they avoid doing any kind of work online. It's so easy to get sucked into spending hours on the computer, one search leading to another or becoming involved in a round of instant messages that fail to offer the depth of true communication or intimacy but that somehow end up taking hours of your time. You can even enlist the help of a buddy who will change your passwords for you and not release them until an agreed-upon time, forcing you to cut back.

At the very least, if you are concerned about getting adequate sleep and optimal rest, consider an *electronic curfew:* no cell phone, TV, or computer an hour before bedtime. In addition to the stress of thinking about work or dealing with electronic demands, the flickering light behind the electronic screen cues your brain to stay awake—the very opposite of the winding-down, preparing-for-sleep message that invites your parasympathetic nervous system to take over. Once you've broken the electronic habit, you may be surprised by how many new ways you find to relax!

Making a Safe Place for Yourself

Our home is supposed to be a safe haven, a place for rest and restoration. Ideally, there would be at least one comforting place in our home that immediately cued the parasympathetic nervous system to take over, allowing the day's stress to melt away and relaxation to begin.

For far too many of us, however, home is simply an extension of the day's stress, a place where we feel even more keenly our 24-hour availability to our children, partner, relatives, friends, and community obligations. A family member's phone call, a colleague's e-mail, a child's question—these may feel constant and inescapable, along with the noise of the television, the pile of waiting work, and a dozen other unrelenting demands.

Many of us are introverts who need to retreat into ourselves to regain our energy. And even the most outer-directed extrovert might need some quiet downtime during a long and stressful day.

If you grew up in a household where you also felt at risk—where your privacy was not respected or where adults' anger, illness, or addictions created a constant sense of potential danger in your life—then it's even more important for you to have a truly safe and controllable space in your own home. Here are a few suggestions for how you might create that safe haven:

- *Arrange the furniture so that your back is never to the door.* Many people feel much more secure and in control when they know that, as soon as the door opens, they can see at a glance who is there.

- *Create one place where you have complete control over the environment.* This may take some ingenuity in a small home, especially if you have children, but you'll be modeling healthy behavior. Both you and your children should be able to say, even if only for a few minutes a day, "I just need a little time for myself right now. I love you, and I'll be there in a few minutes." One way to help your children understand this concept is to choose a time when another responsible adult is home and give your children a kitchen timer with the instruction to wait until the bell rings before coming to get you. Start with just a few minutes, and work up to a half hour or more.

- *Put things in your private space that remind you of your best self.* What makes you happy? What makes you feel good about yourself? What reminds you of who you really are? Find the photographs, objects, and images that bring you back to yourself. Surround yourself with these talismans of your best self.

- *Draw on the relaxing properties of scent.* The sense of smell can reach your emotions at a deeper level than any of the other four senses. Since lavender is so relaxing, consider natural lavender-scented candles, incense, and room fragrances, or perhaps fragrant fresh flowers, to create a restorative atmosphere in your safe space.

- *Use music to unwind.* Classical music, sacred choral music, and other types of relaxing sounds can help you feel safe and at peace.

Quiet Your Mind

If you can find a way to quiet your mind periodically, you can release an enormous amount of stress. One of the most wonderful ways to quiet your mind is through meditation. Meditation offers many health benefits, improving blood pressure, circulation, and heart health; and it also supports mood, self-confidence, and relaxation. It's good for calming anxiety, decreasing muscle tension, and preventing headaches. There is even some evidence that it boosts immune function, helps in post-op healing, reduces premenstrual symptoms, and generally creates a sense of well-being.

Many people find it helpful to take a class in meditation, but you can also practice on your own. Here are three approaches you might enjoy:

- *Mindfulness meditation.* Sit in a comfortable position, ideally in a quiet, peaceful place, with your back straight and your head level. Sit in a chair or on a couch with good back support, or you can make yourself comfortable on the floor or even sitting up in bed, so long as you are sitting up straight, not slouched or reclining. You want the energy to move freely, from the base of your spine right up to the crown of your head. Your eyes may be open or closed. Set a timer for five or ten minutes so that you can relax without checking the time.

Focus your attention on your breathing, becoming aware of each breath. Imagine thoughts passing through your mind and floating away again. If your attention begins to wander, focus on your breathing. It sometimes helps to count each breath, counting to ten and then beginning again. Just breathe and notice what arises.

- *Moving meditation.* You don't have to sit still to meditate. You can take a walk in a beautiful natural spot, or in the city on your lunch hour. You can even do a moving meditation in a crowded, noisy spot, such as a mall, though it may be more challenging. The important thing is to allow your mind to become quiet.

  Set a timer to alert yourself when it's time to head back. Then simply walk at a brisk but comfortable pace. The energy you create in your body will help relieve your stress, while the rest you are giving your mind will create more mental energy. Allow your mind to focus simply on the experience of moving. Notice how your body feels moving through space, how your feet lift and return to the ground, how your back holds you upright, how your hips propel you forward. Pay attention to your movement in as much detail as you can, and tune out the outside world. Alternately, you can move while focusing on your breath, noticing each inhale and exhale; or you can count your breaths, going from one to ten and beginning again. If your mind is focusing on movement, breathing, or counting, it won't be able to return to a worrying or anxious groove, and you'll give your parasympathetic nervous system a chance to kick in.

- *Dance It Out.* I've borrowed this one from the popular TV show *Grey's Anatomy,* in which the stressed-out surgeons try to let go of their romantic and professional problems by "dancing it out." Put on some music you like in a private space, and just dance! Allow yourself to become absorbed by the music, the physical energy, and the sheer joy of moving your body. Just one song's worth of dancing can put you into a different mood for the rest of the day.

ADRENAL-FRIENDLY ACTIVITIES:
WAYS TO BEGIN TO HEAL

- Put a few Post-it notes around your home and work space that remind you to *just breathe.* Try putting one on the receiver of every phone and by your computer.

- Once a day—or even once a week—step outside and take five deep breaths.

- Write yourself a prescription to say *"No."* Use it the next time someone asks you to do something you'd really rather not do. Imagine that I, your health-care practitioner, or someone else concerned with your well-being, has prescribed this *no* for you—and then use the time to do something that makes you happy.

- If you find it difficult to prepare healthy food for yourself, consider picking up your dinner at the grocery store (many places have prepared-food counters) or even having a local caterer deliver your meals. However, be mindful where you shop, since so many prepared foods are overloaded with salt, sugar, unhealthy fats, additives, and artificial ingredients.

- Take a page from the book of Norman Cousins, the American journalist who healed his cancer by watching funny movies, and give yourself time to do something that makes you laugh out loud.

- Whether or not you are traditionally religious, offer up a prayer of gratitude for being alive right now. Take a deep breath; hold it a moment, then exhale. Do it a second time, giving thanks for the ability to breathe in and out, having the breath of life.

- Make some quiet time for yourself—time free from busyness—to get in touch with your spiritual side. You might attend a formal religious event, sit quietly in a peaceful place, or read an inspiring passage or poem. Whether or not you are traditionally religious, you will benefit from taking some time to consider the deeper meaning of your life, rather than simply rushing from task to task.

Be Gentle with Yourself

It took Madison only a few months to reverse her adrenal dysfunction, which was still in the *mild* stage. But by the time she was ready to stop seeing me, she had begun to realize that she had a longer journey ahead of her: unearthing and coming to terms with the buried emotions from her past. When she let up on some of her intense activity, the rage, sorrow, and bewilderment that she had felt since childhood finally caught up with her, and she started looking for help to cope with these new emotional discoveries.

To her own surprise, Madison had discovered a real love of movement that her rigorous exercise schedule had only partially satisfied. She began taking a modern-dance class and also started seeing a dance therapist I recommended, who used movement as a means to work through the remains of Madison's childhood pain.

We'll look more deeply at this type of emotional work in Chapter 9. I want to leave you with one of the most moving examples I know that demonstrates how profoundly our lifestyle choices can affect our health. Researchers measured the levels of T3 and T4 helper cells—key components of the immune system—among a group of medical students. Then half the group was shown a movie of a simulated rape, while the other half was shown a movie about Mother Teresa. Afterward, researchers measured the helper cells again. Those who had seen the rape had lower levels of the helper cells, while those who had seen the more optimistic vision of humanity had increased immune function.

If this was the effect of students watching *other* people being treated with violence or compassion, how much greater is the effect of your own self-treatment and self-talk? When you speak to yourself lovingly—in your internal dialogue and via your own actions— you help to heal yourself, literally giving yourself a kind of loving medicine. If I leave you with just one thought from this chapter, it is to be gentle with yourself, to go at your own pace, and to salute yourself for doing just as much as you can—and no more.

chapter
eight

HEALING YOURSELF

As a health-care provider, I find it most exciting that the body has the capacity to heal itself. Although many of us tend to become somewhat fatalistic about our health, we can actually transform our physical, mental, and emotional condition once we understand how these aspects of our being are related. So I'd like to share with you two key reasons for feeling optimistic, empowered, and motivated to change:

- *We can alter many of our body's responses—even if we're genetically "programmed" in a certain way.* In the past few years, there have been a lot of news stories about genetic predisposition to certain diseases, particularly diabetes, heart disease, and cancer. Due to our experience in the womb, we may also be born with a tendency to gain or retain weight. These predispositions and tendencies are the "givens" that apparently we can't change.

    Yet there is a great deal of science to support the notion that we *can* change how these tendencies express themselves. If you feed your body the right food and nutrients, and if you choose a healthy lifestyle that includes exercise and mindfulness, you can do a great deal to ensure that certain genes—particularly the ones for heart disease, diabetes, and many types of cancer—never get expressed. You can also reprogram your body to overcome its prenatal experience, rewriting your metabolism and making it easier for you to maintain a healthy weight.

- *The mind, emotions, and spirit have an enormous impact on the body.* How we think and feel about ourselves and the world, and how we experience a spiritual connection, can make a huge difference when it comes to healing the body. If we're prisoners of our past, responding with amygdala-driven impulsiveness to replay the same panic, anxiety, sorrow, or anger that colored our past, our bodies will find it far more difficult to heal. But if we learn—through the techniques that I'll share with you in Chapter 9—to reprogram our emotional responses, our bodies can begin to shake off the burdens of the past.

How exciting and empowering is that? Just by the choices we make each day about what we eat and how we live, we can alter the way our genes express themselves and create our own good health.

These are not simply articles of faith. There's a great deal of science supporting both of these points—and in this chapter, I'll share it with you.

Conducting Your Genetic "Chorus"

In recent years, a lot of research has come out about our genes and the myriad ways they affect our minds, bodies, and personalities. Scientists have discovered that many of us are born with a predisposition to certain disorders, such as diabetes, heart disease, some types of cancer, and some autoimmune conditions.

For many of my patients, this is depressing news. They've begun to think of their genes as dooming them to an unhealthy life, predicting an inevitable decline into a predetermined illness.

"How can I fight my own genes?" my patient Nora asked me one day. "My mother has rheumatoid arthritis, my grandmother has rheumatoid arthritis—and now you're telling me that in addition to all the other things going wrong with me, I'm at risk for that, too. Clearly, there's a genetic problem here—so what are we supposed to do about it?"

Like many of us, Nora was thinking of her genes as a given, a set of instructions that programmed her for life. But as I told her, the process is far more dynamic and variable than that, with lots of opportunities for intervention. New discoveries in *epigenetics*— the effect of mechanisms other than DNA on genetic expression—show that while we may be born with certain tendencies, the way we live is often a deciding factor in how those tendencies play out. One key aspect of epigenetics is *nutrigenomics:* the effect of nutrition on our genetic expression, which means that what we eat can have a profound impact on our bodies and brains.

Instead of thinking of your genes as fixed and given, I invite you to think of them as voices in a chorus. Some of the voices are loud and clear, some are muffled, and some are virtually silent. And the way we conduct that chorus has a great deal to do with which voices are lowered and which ones ring out.

Nora, for example, might well have been born with a genetic tendency to rheumatoid arthritis, which is an autoimmune condition. But, as we have seen, a stressful life—one with too little time spent in "parasympathetic mode"—puts a strain on our adrenals and our immune system. Because there's so much cross talk between the HPA axis and our body's other systems, an overworked HPA axis might well trigger autoimmune problems that would otherwise have lain dormant, encouraging the "autoimmune" part of Nora's genetic code to scream at the top of its lungs.

By the same token, calming and healing the HPA axis could help quiet the genes that were predisposing Nora to a disorder. Altering her relationship to stress and beginning an anti-inflammatory, adrenal-friendly diet might help quiet that troubling part of Nora's genetic code, reducing or even ending her symptoms. Nora may always have an underlying tendency to develop rheumatoid arthritis. But she can either muffle that tendency or turn up its volume—the choice is hers.

You may have read about Morgan Spurlock, creator of the documentary *Super Size Me.* As part of his experiment, Spurlock ate nothing but fast food from McDonald's for 30 days and filmed himself gaining weight. Interestingly, Spurlock had been in above-average physical condition before beginning the project, but his unhealthy diet not only packed on the pounds, it also created a toxic liver and many other severe complications. Only after months of effort was Spurlock able to return to his previous state of health.

Yet when Swedish researcher Fredrik Nyström repeated the experiment with a group of student volunteers at Linköping University, his students had quite different results. Though some students did gain weight, others stayed the same, and still others even built muscle. No one gained weight as fast as Spurlock had, and they avoided the liver damage and other extreme side effects that he suffered.

Why did Spurlock respond so differently? Nyström speculates that his previous vegetarian diet may have affected his ability to metabolize the fast food—one version of how our diet affects our body's responses. I wonder, too, whether Spurlock's own genetic code—his liver's inborn vulnerability to a high-fat diet—had simply never been challenged before. Perhaps when Spurlock ate the kinds of foods that muffled his genetic tendency to insulin resistance, his body functioned well. When he stressed his system with an unhealthy diet, he came down with numerous symptoms and felt horrible—even though another group of young people was able to eat the very same diet with relatively few short-term effects.

To me, both the Spurlock experiment and the Swedish experiment are eloquent testimony to our own power to influence our genetic expression. How exciting to have such power over our own health! We may not be able to choose the members of our genetic chorus. But we can have a great deal of choice in which voices are silenced and which are heard.

Where the Music Begins

Epigenetics—the conducting of our genetic chorus—begins in the womb. If your mother had a stressful life, and especially if she faced a shortage of food or dieted strenuously during her pregnancy with you, your cells learned that they had better prepare for a high-stress life and hang on to every calorie. Accordingly, you turned up the volume on your tendency to retain weight and perhaps also cued your HPA axis to work on a hair trigger. Before you were even born, you were creating your genetic chorus, perhaps programming a tendency to hold on to weight or to react intensely to stress.

This was certainly the case with Nora. Her grandmother had grown up in difficult conditions, enduring dire poverty in rural Maine. Her great-grandmother had barely enough to eat when she was carrying Nora's grandmother. As a result, Nora's grandmother developed a tendency to retain weight, conserving every calorie against hard times to come.

Nora's grandmother, however, had adequate access to food—and so her prenatal programming, rather than saving her from famine, cued her to become overweight. Interestingly, Nora's great-aunt, who was also conceived and born during difficult times, never developed a weight problem. The interaction between genes and our prenatal environment is a dynamic one, and there's a lot we don't yet understand about it. But just as Morgan Spurlock had one reaction to his fast-food diet while the Swedish students had differing results, so did Nora's grandmother and great-aunt have two different responses to their prenatal diet.

Meanwhile, Nora's grandmother passed on that epigenetic pattern—that tendency to retain weight—to Nora's mother, who passed it on to Nora. As a result, three generations of women have struggled with their weight.

Nora's experience was reproduced on a large scale during the Dutch *Hongerwinter*, that brutal winter of 1944–1945 when the Nazi-controlled Netherlands were completely cut off from any access to food. Some 30,000 people starved to death, while the survivors were reduced to official rations of 400 to 800 calories a day. Consider that most adults need 2,000 calories per day and pregnant or nursing mothers need 2,300 calories, and you can see how dire the situation was.

Nevertheless, nearly 40,000 babies were born that winter—an extraordinary testament to how determined our bodies are to create and preserve life even under the most desperate circumstances. Two decades later, researchers began to study what had happened to these children of famine. What they found is further evidence of the power of epigenetics.

Not surprisingly, fetuses that had been in their last trimesters during the worst of the famine were born with low birth weights. Later, as more food became available, they grew up as normal children, with no outward sign of those difficult years. As adults, however, those same children suffered from very high rates of diabetes. Their blood-sugar regulation had been disrupted in the womb, setting them up for potential lifelong problems.

Some parents conceived children during the famine but had normal access to food in their final trimester. Those babies were of normal birth weight when they were born— apparently they had been able to "catch up" during the last three months of pregnancy. However, when they grew up and had their own children, their babies were unusually small. Their prenatal experience of famine had taught their genes that food would always be scarce, and their genetic chorus changed as a result.

Moreover, the girls who had been conceived during the famine suffered from significantly higher rates of midlife diabetes and obesity. Their genetic choruses—and in some cases, their children's genetic choruses as well—were altered. Even though only one generation experienced the famine directly, three generations showed the results.

What if the children of the "hunger winter" had been given diets and exercise plans designed to redirect the programming they had received before they were born? What if they had tried to "reconduct" their genetic choruses, using diet and lifestyle choices to turn up the volume on some genes while muffling others?

We'll never know. What we do know is that when Nora began her own adrenal-friendly diet and exercise plan, she was able to reverse a three-generation pattern in her own family, getting down to her ideal weight and remaining there. Thousands of my patients can tell similar stories. Making healthy, self-loving decisions about diet and lifestyle can overcome both genetic tendencies and prenatal experience to create the joyous choruses of our choice.

Stress—and Its Antidote

Just as hunger in the womb programs our bodies to retain weight, stress in the womb sets us up for trouble with the HPA axis. Stressing a rat in pregnancy, for example, causes lifelong changes in the offspring—including increased anxiety. Stressing a human child also has dramatic results—extreme stress can prevent a child from growing.

Our genetic chorus may be programmed in the womb, but our bodies are reprogrammed throughout our lives. If you had a rough beginning but a safe, secure childhood with lots of hugs and nutritious foods, your HPA axis learned to calm down. You saved the high production of stress hormones for situations that were truly challenging, the ones that genuinely required a fight-or-flight response.

If, on the other hand, you grew up in a family with lots of yelling, a great deal of insecurity, a parent who was chronically ill, or other major stressors, you learned to keep your HPA axis turned up. When every day brings a potential emergency, it's important to have your stress hormones at the ready, flowing freely into your body at the slightest provocation.

For example, Katie, the restaurateur we met in Chapter 2, had grown up with a loud, angry father. Every time Katie came home from school, she went into hyperalert mode. Was this going to be a "yelling day," or was he in a good mood? Was this one of those days when she should avoid him, or would it be all right to start a conversation, maybe even to climb onto his lap for a hug? For Katie, knowing that her father's mood could change on a dime meant that no time was ever really safe. Whether or not her father was actually yelling, Katie learned to watch his mood every moment and to be on alert.

As a result, Katie's body became accustomed to high levels of stress hormones that only rarely declined. Her childhood experience modified her genetic chorus, her patterns of behavior, and her emotional expectations. But she absolutely has the power to reverse those patterns and rewrite the music for her genetic chorus. And she needs to give herself credit for even beginning to change.

Significantly, treating ourselves with anger and criticism helps keep our stress levels high, while treating ourselves with love and care can help to reverse the whole process. There is a lot of science on this, too, showing that love, nurturance, and care can make an enormous difference to our health. For example, scientists have been fascinated by the comparison of two post–World War II German orphanages, which were identical as far as diet, doctors' visits, and other types of care. One was run by a warm, loving woman who played with the children and comforted them when they cried. The other was run by a woman who had as little to do with the children as possible and who frequently criticized them, usually in front of the whole group. The children under the care of the warm, loving matron literally grew faster and gained more weight than the other children, even though they were all given the same kinds of food and medical care. Love enabled one group of children to thrive, even as lack of love stunted the other children's growth.

This wasn't just coincidence. When the cold, critical matron left her post, she was replaced by the warm, loving woman from the other orphanage. Right away, the children under the care of the loving woman began to gain in height and weight, while the children she had left behind began to grow more slowly.

These results have been confirmed on an individual level with numerous children. When taken out of abusive, neglectful, or otherwise stressful environments and given warm, nurturing care, they begin to grow at a more rapid rate. Almost more dramatically, the results have also been confirmed in animal studies. When baby rats are separated from their mothers, for example, growth stops. What makes it start again? It's not the mother's smell, which scientists confirmed by pumping that smell into the rats' cages. It's not passive contact with the mother either—allowing baby rats to be near the mother when she was anesthetized made no difference at all. What does seem to matter is active touch, the physical expression of love. If human researchers mimicked the mother's active licking by stroking the baby rats in the right pattern, the babies' growth resumed. Other studies have shown that handling baby rats makes them grow faster and larger.

Perhaps the most dramatic animal studies in this field were conducted by Harry Harlow, a University of Wisconsin researcher who wanted to determine once and for all why infants are attached to their mothers. When he was conducting his studies in the 1950s and 1960s, many scientists insisted that Mother was valuable for the functions she performed and the needs she fulfilled, primarily that she relieved her children's hunger. Love, they thought, had nothing to do with it—people simply wanted to ensure that their body's needs were met.

Harlow didn't agree. So he raised infant rhesus monkeys without mothers, giving them a choice of two artificial surrogates. One had a wooden monkey head and a wire mesh torso with a milk bottle stuck in it. If the reason to love mother was because she gave food, that would be the surrogate to choose. The other also had a wooden head and wire mesh torso—but that torso was wrapped in terry cloth, soft and comforting to snuggle in, though there was no milk bottle. Yet the comfort-giving terry-cloth mother was the one that the monkey babies chose. Even the illusion of love was preferable, it seemed—the need for love was stronger even than hunger.

The animal studies are echoed in a similar experiment conducted with premature infants in neonatology wards. When a team of researchers held the preemies for 15 minutes, three times a day, they grew nearly 50 percent faster, matured faster behaviorally, and were generally more active and alert. They were released from the hospital nearly a week sooner than premature infants who were not touched, and they continued to do better months after they were released.

Think about that for a moment. A loving touch made an enormous difference in the health of babies who were facing huge challenges as soon as they were born. They were weak, small, and premature, but human touch—love—helped them to thrive.

There's the science behind my heartfelt request to you: Surround yourself with as much love as you can, from as many people in your life as possible. Hug your children, your partner, and your friends, and let them hug you. Even if your love is expressed over long distances—by phone or e-mail—stay in regular contact with the people you care about. Allow yourself to feel their love for you and your love for them.

Treat yourself lovingly as well. Think of yourself as a child who needs to be soothed, comforted, and given treats. Nurture yourself the way that warm, loving matron at the German orphanage cared for her charges, and watch yourself grow and thrive as a result. Loving treatment is good for your morale. It's good for your weight. And it's good for your health. Speaking as a health-care practitioner, I know there is no better medicine.

Be Good to Yourself

As we've seen, the way you treat yourself can make an enormous difference in how your body, mind, and spirit respond. Changing your internal conversation is one key way to turn down the stress and turn up the relaxation. I've struggled with these issues, too, and I know how hard it can be to create a new conversation. The key is practice. Every time you catch yourself being mean to yourself, stop, interrupt yourself, and choose a different response. The same goes with your diet, exercise plan, and all other aspects of self-care. Finding a way to do them lovingly, rather than self-critically ("I'm so fat!" "I'm so lazy!" "I'm so undisciplined!") is a crucial part of reversing chronic stress.

Our ultimate goal is to treat ourselves with love and respect, providing our bodies, minds, emotions, and spirits with the care and nurturing that they need. If at the moment that sounds too challenging, let's take it down a notch. Just notice how you talk to and treat yourself. Then, if you have the opportunity, interrupt yourself whenever you hear the mean or overly critical inner monologue and choose a different response.

SIGNS OF SELF-LOVE

"How do I know when I'm loving myself?" That's what one patient actually asked me, which got me thinking. Here's my list of some signs of self-love. Can you think of others?

I know I love myself when:

- I start making time for myself.

- I say no to additional duties and pressures and set up boundaries to protect myself.

- I forgive myself—not just for the trivial mistakes, but for the big ones, too.

- I let go of some unrealistic expectations of myself and feel good about what I have accomplished.

- I find one thing to do each day that makes me truly happy—even if it's as brief as smelling a flower on my kitchen table or enjoying the feel of body lotion after my shower.

- I chew and really taste my food.

- I take a moment to breathe deeply and savor the breath.

- When I hear myself think something demeaning about myself, I push the pause button, rewind the tape, and put in a new tape that's more compassionate.

- I take an "electronic Sabbath" for an hour, a day, a weekend—no computers, no cell phones, and nothing work-related.

Adrenal-Friendly Dos and Don'ts

Here are a few concrete suggestions for how you might begin:

- DO take a self-inventory to identify your "critics" and come up with some positive, nurturing messages to replace the harsh ones. We all have those voices in our heads—the ones we created after listening to our mother, our father, our teachers, maybe an older brother or sister—the voices telling us we're not good enough, not smart enough, not pretty enough, not enough. The people who spoke to us as children probably had no idea how powerful their words would be—but here we are, years later, repeating those same old criticisms to ourselves and reliving the hurt again and again. Identifying these voices and figuring out where they come from takes away a great deal of their power. Creating supportive messages to replace the critical ones can do wonders for our physical as well as our emotional health. (I'll offer specific suggestions for taking this step in Chapter 9.)

- DO commit to asking for and accepting help. Many of us feel the entire world resting upon our shoulders. Even if we have supportive friends or an active partner, we still tend to feel the major responsibility for the household, the family, the community, the tasks at work, and that there's no one to whom we can delegate, no one on whom we can lean. If you recognize yourself in this description, start to break the pattern. Identify people—friends, family, loved ones, colleagues—on whom you can rely and start asking for and accepting their help. You'll feel better—and your health will show the difference.

- DO notice who in your life is truly helpful and supportive—and who is not. Sometimes, when we become aware of our internal critics, we realize that some of the people around us are echoing those voices and supporting our most negative self-image. If you're starting to see that those around you don't truly support you, it may be time to make some changes. You deserve a support system of caring people who see you as valuable and lovable, and who always leave you feeling better about yourself. If this is not true of many of the people in your life, it may be time to make some changes in your support system.

- DO commit to making time for your own needs. Would you be surprised to learn that taking 15 minutes a day to do "nothing" might be the best thing you could ever do for your health? Would you be surprised to learn that for many of my patients—and maybe even for you, too—it's the hardest to follow of all my suggestions? If you can't take 15, take 5. If you can't take 5, take a minute—60 seconds—that is all about you, you, you. I promise, your adrenals will be grateful.

- DON'T say anything to yourself that you might not say to a girlfriend. "You're so stupid!" "You're so fat!" "You look awful today!" "Why can't you do anything right?" Would you speak that way to anyone, let alone someone you cared about? No? Then why talk that way to yourself? This only adds to your adrenal stress load, which will definitely make you feel worse.

- DON'T make your diet a punishment. Eat foods that are really delicious and that you really enjoy. You don't have to live on raw celery and bean sprouts—there are plenty of healthy but delectable choices. (I've offered specific meal plans in Chapter 6.)

- DON'T push yourself too hard. Exercise is good for you—but if you're suffering from severe or even moderate adrenal dysfunction, the wrong kind of exercise can make your poor adrenals feel even more stressed. If vigorous workouts leave you energized and refreshed, they are helping you to improve your health. But if your exercise routine leaves you feeling exhausted, choose something less strenuous: a leisurely bike ride, a slow swim, even a 20-minute stroll. Many of my patients protest that they have the willpower and discipline to push through the exhaustion, but that's part of the problem: if your adrenals aren't functioning properly, pushing them harder will only make things worse. What you're looking for is not more stress but a balanced, gentle approach to exercise. (I've offered specific exercise plans in Chapter 7.)

Change Is Possible

As we conclude this chapter, I'd like to leave you with the words of Columbia University psychiatrist and researcher Norman Doidge, author of *The Brain That Changes Itself.* Doidge stated at a recent neuroscience conference, "The plasticity of the brain is the most important scientific discovery in the past 400 years." As Hoffman Institute president Raz Ingrasci commented, "Why is this such an important discovery? Because it means that we can grow and change throughout our life span. Change is not only possible; it is an aspect of the structure of our brain."

In other words, our brains were meant to change, and that means that they *can* change. And once we change our brains, it's only a small next step to change our bodies—and our lives.

ADRENAL-FRIENDLY ACTIVITIES:
WAYS TO BEGIN TO HEAL

- *A friendly connection.* Choose one friend who always makes you feel better about yourself. Find some way to be in contact with this person at least three times a week, even if it's only a brief e-mail, a quick text, or a five-minute phone call. Consider telling this friend that you're making some changes to improve your health, and that you've decided that being in touch is actually going to make you healthier. If you can't imagine finding the time to call or e-mail your friend, ask if he or she would be willing to leave you brief phone messages or send short e-mails or texts a few times a week for the next 30 days.

- *A loving touch.* Ask your partner or a loving friend to give you at least one ten-minute massage each week. You can do this fully clothed, in the midst of other activities; but find a quiet, private space in which you can allow yourself to relax. Just having someone work on your shoulders, your spine, and your lower back can help you release stress and signal your parasympathetic nervous system to begin the relaxation process. You can also have someone massage your hands and arms—especially good if you spend a lot of time on the computer—or, for a real treat, he or she can work on your feet. If you have the time and money, consider getting a professional massage—perhaps even once a week.

- *A bit of pampering.* Splurge on a manicure, a pedicure, or both! Consider getting the kind where you also receive a foot, leg, or shoulder massage. Perhaps stopping by the salon once a week or once every other week can become part of your routine—a moment to breathe, shift into "parasympathetic mode," and allow yourself to be taken care of.

- *What makes you happy?* Take five minutes and jot down as quickly as possible a list of all the things that make you truly happy. Don't stop to think—simply write whatever comes to mind. A hug from your kids? A fragrant rose by your bedside? The smell of the ocean? The taste of fresh strawberries? Put your list somewhere at home or at work where you'll see it every day and then allow yourself one minute each day to envision one item on that list. For "extra credit," actually give yourself that item.

EMOTIONAL
WORK

At first glance, Jenna seemed like a shy, mousy woman, the kind of person whom
you'd easily overlook at a party or a meeting. A public-interest lawyer, she worked hard
for her clients, who thought the world of her, but most of the people who knew her
didn't realize the significance of the contribution she made to their lives.

At age 36, Jenna had two children, a girl in middle school and a boy who was just
starting high school. She was a devoted volunteer at both their schools, and because
her husband's job as a pilot often took him out of town, most of the chauffeuring and
homework monitoring fell to her.

As if this didn't keep her busy enough, Jenna had a circle of friends who had all
come to count on her. If you had to go to the hospital for a procedure, Jenna was the
one you asked to sit with you in the waiting room, to hold your hand and help you
cope. If you had just gotten dumped by your new love interest or had a horrible fight
with your partner, Jenna was the one you called for advice. If you were struggling with
a major career change, confused about a life choice, or just feeling blue and discouraged, Jenna was the friend with the best advice, the staunchest support, and the most
reliable comfort.

As a result, Jenna was suffering from a severe case of adrenal dysfunction. A Workhorse, she dragged herself out of bed every morning, relied on coffee and diet sodas to make it through her day, and then stayed up every night, wired and tired, trying to come down from her late-night "cortisol high." Every night, she told me, she found it difficult to sleep because her mind was racing with thoughts of her clients, her children, her husband, and her friends: what did they need, what did they want, how could she help them?

"It sounds as though you're a wonderful support to everyone in your life," I said carefully. "But where is the room for Jenna?"

As we talked, it soon became clear that even when Jenna did manage to take time for herself, she almost always felt guilty about it. But she was quite resistant to looking at her emotions and at her emotional history. She was willing to change her diet, take the supplements I suggested, and make time for some gentle exercise. At my suggestion, she even enrolled in a yoga class and added 15 minutes to her schedule for morning meditation. But when I asked her to look at her childhood history and how it might relate to her habit of saying yes to everyone but herself, she balked.

"I love my friends and my family, and they need me," she insisted. "That's why I say yes—not for some childhood thing. And my clients and my kids' schools—they need me, too."

As I had warned her, though, the diet, exercise, and lifestyle suggestions took Jenna only so far. Her anxiety, sleep problems, and perimenopausal symptoms continued, and while she lost some weight, she was nowhere near her goal.

I think what really opened Jenna to doing the emotional work was coming into her daughter Olivia's room one night and finding her in tears. When Jenna questioned Olivia, she learned that her daughter hadn't yet been able to start the next day's homework assignment because she had been on the phone all night with first one friend, then another, helping them with their problems while neglecting her own work. Now it was bedtime and Olivia was exhausted. But when Jenna insisted that Olivia get some sleep, Olivia became even more distraught. "It's for Ms. Ewell's class," she kept saying. "She's so nice. She'll be so disappointed."

Jenna appreciated that Olivia wanted to get her work done, but she was also concerned about her daughter. So she suggested that Olivia do only the main portion of the assignment and let go of the extra-credit portion she had planned to do. If anything, Olivia's distress increased. "But it's for Ms. *Ewell*," she wailed. "It has to be *perfect*."

To Jenna's dismay, Olivia seemed to be taking on many of Jenna's own stresses and strains. Our children watch what we do, not what we say. Seeing her daughter exhaust herself for the sake of others made Jenna realize that her own frantic round of activity was not only depleting herself, it was teaching her daughter to do likewise. Still reluctant but now also determined to make some changes, she spoke to her therapist about being ready to start EMDR (eye movement desensitization and reprocessing), an integrated mind-body approach to therapy that I describe later in this chapter.

Working with her EMDR therapist, Jenna came to realize that her deep-seated need to care for others had its roots in her childhood where, because of an impoverished family in which her father worked two jobs and her mother was a night-shift waitress, Jenna had become a caretaker at a very young age. Of course, Jenna was a genuinely loving and caring person, and she sincerely wanted to do her best for her clients, family, and friends. But there was a driven, compulsive quality to her activities, a sense that she *couldn't* say no and that she was putting herself and others in danger if she ever took time for herself. This might indeed have been true for the ten-year-old girl with two overworked parents, but it was no longer true for the adult woman with a network of friends and family that was willing and able to support *her.*

As she came to terms with these childhood wounds, Jenna began to blossom in unexpected ways. Not only did she give up some of her activities and say no occasionally to her loved ones, she actually started dressing in a more colorful and attractive manner, and began to speak up more at social occasions. It was as if she were finally feeling entitled to take up space and be noticed, to care for herself and see herself as beautiful. By working on her childhood baggage, Jenna transformed both her feelings and her caretaking role—and relief from adrenal symptoms was only one of her rewards.

Physical Approaches to the Pain of the Past

If you have adrenal dysfunction, you are almost by definition living with some form of chronic stress—environmental, physical, situational, emotional, or some combination thereof. If any portion of your stress comes from your situation or your emotions—and it almost always does!—you might want to consider whether you could lessen your allostatic load by getting rid of some of your emotional baggage.

As we've seen throughout this book, our response to stressful circumstances is rarely based in the present alone. Far more often, if we have strong feelings of anxiety, irritation, frustration, sorrow, or guilt, we are reacting at least partially to the pains of childhood, acting out the difficulties in our childhood relationship with our parents. Katie, whom we met in Chapter 2, brought her childhood anxieties about her father's anger to her adult relationship with her husband. Madison, whom we met in Chapter 7, carried into adulthood her childhood responses to her father's absences and her mother's obsession with weight. And Jenna, whom we met at the beginning of this chapter, was not only acting out her childhood fears of not being able to live up to her overwhelming responsibility, she was also passing those fears on to her daughter.

So how do we free ourselves from these prisons of the past? Many of us turn to various forms of talk therapy to gain some understanding of the patterns that are getting in our way. In my experience, traditional talk therapy can be a fabulous stepping-stone to transformation, but it may not reach us at the deepest places in our bodies, where our emotional memories live. Talk therapy brings us awareness of our patterns and extraordinary insight into some of the reasons for our responses. But to truly alter those responses, we often have to go to a place deeper than words, working on a more physical and emotional level than the experience of simply talking.

Many of my patients have discovered possibilities for self-transformation and "emotional reprogramming" in approaches that are based on unlocking the deep connections between mind, body, emotions, and spirit, at a level that "just talking" often fails to reach. As Candace Pert has shown in her groundbreaking *Molecules of Emotion,* we now understand that much of the pain from the past is often literally stored in our tissue, formed before we have words or conscious awareness of what's happening. As a result, the following techniques can help to address buried emotional pain.

Consider whether one of the following approaches might help you connect more deeply to yourself and help you to unlock that pain:

- *Chiropractic.* This discipline is based on the premise that a host of ills can result from the misalignment of the spine, which causes pressure on surrounding tissue as well as disrupts the healthy flow of *neurotransmitters* (biochemicals that regulate brain function and mood). Chiropractic has been shown to have significant benefits to both mind and body, including helping people to overcome addiction and alleviating anxiety and depression. If emotional memories are locked within your body, chiropractic may help to liberate your childhood pain as well as relieve your spine, especially if you are also doing some form of talk therapy or emotional work at the same time. (For more information, see http://nccam.nih.gov/health/chiropractic/.)

- *Feldenkrais.* The Feldenkrais Method of Somatic Education was founded by Russian-born physicist and engineer Moshe Feldenkrais, who developed it out of his studies of martial arts in order to overcome his own chronic physical pain. The method includes group Awareness Through Movement classes and individual Functional Integration Lessons, both of which are designed to encourage you to learn to move more naturally and with less energy, and eventually, to broaden your self-image by expanding your range of movement. Since, as we have seen, the body holds memories of traumatic events, freeing yourself from rigid patterns of movement could help free you from rigid ideas as well. (For more information, see www.feldenkrais.com.)

- *Guided imagery.* Harnessing the imagination to create a vision of reality can help us transform our lives. Guided imagery can involve visualization as well as tapping into sounds, smells, and tactile experiences. Studies show that a biophysical response to positive imagery can effectively override the hardwiring of engrained thought patterns and habits to help create better health and attain otherwise unreachable goals. (For more information, see http://belleruthnaparstek.com and http://healthjourneys.com.)

- *Hypnosis or self-hypnosis.* A technique that creates an altered state of consciousness, hypnotherapy can be self-administered or done through the help of a practitioner. Hypnotherapy can be effective in behavior modification, such as to stop smoking or end compulsive eating; as well as to treat trauma, phobia, and pain. (For more information, see www.natboard.com.)

- *Polarity therapy.* This form of hands-on therapy works with your body's electromagnetic field to regulate the flow and balance of your energy. The approach identifies and frees places where energy is blocked, unbalanced, or "frozen" into a fixed pattern. Developed by naturopath, chiropractor, and osteopath Randolph Stone, polarity therapy identifies a number of factors that affect the human energy field, including diet, environment, movement, touch, attitudes, relationships, trauma, and life experience. As the body's energy is unblocked, your spirit may be released from traumatic events of the past. (For more information, see www.polaritytherapy.org.)

- *The Relaxation Response.* Pioneered by Herbert Benson, a Harvard internist, the relaxation response involves attaining a state of deep relaxation whereby a person can counteract the ill effects of pain, anxiety, and stress. Employing a variety of mind-body exercises to achieve a meditative state, the relaxation response has been used for years to help people successfully overcome all sorts of physiological and psychological problems, including high blood pressure, addiction, and some stress-related infertility issues. (For more information, see www.relaxationresponse.org.)

- *Rolfing.* Named for founder Ida P. Rolf, Rolfing Structural Integration works to release energy stored in the body's *fascia,* or connective tissues, thus relieving stress and alleviating physical pain. By opening up areas of the body that had been previously clenched in tension, Rolfing can potentially help you release experiences that your body is holding tightly and seeking to repress. As your body is realigned and brought into balance, your emotions and spirit may experience a similar relief. (For more information, see www.rolf.org.)

- *Integrative Manual Therapy (IMT).* Developed over the past three decades by Sharon Giammatteo, IMT seeks to address patients' needs in comprehensive and holistic ways, including nutrition, body work, and "body-based psychotherapeutic approaches." Practitioners have addressed a number of disorders using IMT, including attention deficit disorder and chronic fatigue syndrome. Using gentle manipulative techniques, IMT can be used to alleviate physical pain. Then, as we have seen, the physical release may also unlock the bodily centers of emotional distress. (For more information, see www.centerimt.com.)

- *Music therapy.* Have you ever noticed how listening to music seems to reach you at a deep emotional level, opening up feelings whose sources you can't always identify? Music therapy relies on that effect, using your experience of listening to music, writing songs, and performing or improvising music to reach you in places where your rational, verbal self may be unwilling to go. Just as music can unlock emotions and memories, music therapy seeks to free you from emotional baggage of which you may not be consciously aware. (For more information, see www.musictherapy.org.)

- *Art therapy.* Visual expression is another way to bypass our rational selves and reach deep into our emotional histories. Art therapy has been successfully used among people of all ages to address anxiety, depression, and addiction, as well as the after-effects of trauma, violence, and domestic abuse. As we have seen, the emotional pain of childhood may exist in our bodies and our unconscious minds at a level that our cerebral cortex doesn't access. Art therapy can be a way of uncovering and working through that pain. (For more information, see www.arttherapy.org.)

- *Dance and movement therapy.* To quote from the website of the American Dance Therapy Association, ". . . Dance/Movement Therapists mobilize resources from that place within where body and mind are one." What better way to access the hurts and confusions that our bodies hold? Dance therapy can be conducted individually or in a group, with beneficial results for mind, body, emotions, and spirit. "Dancing it out" is not just a metaphor but an accredited way of releasing fears, pain, and trauma while connecting to the joys of movement. (For more information, see www.adta.org.)

- *Pet therapy.* Pet therapy, also known as animal-assisted therapy, relies on animals to produce beneficial side effects such as lowering blood pressure, encouraging socialization, promoting walking, and increasing emotional well-being. Horseback riding has been shown to help with balance and body control. (For more information, see www.healthline.com/galecontent/pet-therapy.)

Emotional Freedom Technique

There are a number of mind-body techniques that go even deeper than the physical approaches I just discussed. One that I personally find fascinating is known as *Emotional Freedom Technique* (EFT). Founded by nondenominational minister Gary Craig, EFT combines some of the insights of mind-body medicine with aspects of acupuncture. As we saw in Chapter 7, acupuncture is an ancient tradition of Chinese medicine based on a theory of *meridians,* or energy pathways. It uses tiny needles to bring healing and relaxation by stimulating these pathways, freeing vital energies to restore your health.

Likewise, in EFT, you tap certain meridian points with your fingertips to rebalance your energy and heal both emotional and physical stress.

If you're interested in EFT, you can find a free instruction manual online, or look online at www.eftuniverse.com. Practitioners recommend undertaking EFT for its emotional benefits as well as its physical ones, and to use it along with some form of traditional therapy.

Since EFT addresses emotional stress—a key source of adrenal dysfunction—I think it has enormous potential for healing the adrenals. I also appreciate that once you learn the basic technique, you can "tap yourself" in key places to alleviate anxiety. I wonder whether the technique helps cue our parasympathetic nervous systems to restore balance, which would make it even more useful in addressing adrenal dysfunction. In any case, though the technique seems very simple, I've seen it produce amazing results.

EMDR: Eye Movement Desensitization and Reprocessing

Like Jenna, many of my patients have had extraordinary success with EMDR, an approach that integrates a number of different types of therapy into a comprehensive mind-body experience. Psychodynamic, cognitive-behavioral, interpersonal, experiential, and body-centered therapies are all part of EMDR, which seeks to release you from the hold of past experiences while helping you to set new, healthier patterns of behavior for the future. What I love about this approach is the way it integrates body, mind, and emotion, at a level that traditional talk therapy rarely achieves.

A key aspect of EMDR is known as "dual stimulation," a fascinating process that can help you reprogram your emotional and mental responses. First, you identify the most vivid visual image that relates to a painful memory, such as the time your father yelled at you for not being ready when he came to pick you up after school. Maybe he called you stupid, inconsiderate, or selfish, leaving you with an anxious feeling about how loved ones would respond to any future mistakes, as well as a set of negative beliefs about yourself. The painful incident would then include both a visual component (your memory), a mental component (your beliefs), and an emotional component (your feelings). Physical sensations (the anxious clenching of your muscles and tightening of your stomach) are also part of the experience.

Next, you are asked to identify a positive belief to replace the old negative one. For example, if your negative belief is, "I'm selfish and inconsiderate, and I always disappoint the people I love," accompanied by a sense of panic or anxiety, your preferred positive belief might be, "I'm loving and generous, and even when I make mistakes, the people I love are happy to have me in their lives." The therapist will work with you to evaluate how accurate both the negative and the positive beliefs are.

After that, you're asked to focus on the image, the negative thought, and the unpleasant bodily sensations while moving your eyes back and forth to follow the therapist's fingers, usually for about 20 or 30 seconds. Sometimes instead of asking you to use your eyes, the therapist may have you focus on sounds or on being gently tapped on the arm. During that time—as you are focusing on both a negative experience from the past and on a sensory experience in the present—you're invited to simply notice whatever happens. Then you're asked to let your mind go blank, and again, simply notice your response.

Eventually, you'll discover that the negative experience has lost its emotional charge. You may remember the incident, but you no longer feel anxious and distressed as you do, and you may not necessarily think, *I'm selfish and inconsiderate* as you remember. At that point, the therapist asks you to think about the positive belief you've identified, to focus yet again on the negative incident you began with, and to repeat once more the eye movements or the experience of listening to tones or being tapped. You continue to share your responses with the therapist, who helps you process the negative thoughts and feelings and emphasize the positive ones.

Eventually, after one or more sessions, you find yourself adapting and having new thoughts and feelings that enable you to respond differently to stressful or painful situations. You may find yourself taking new action to change some difficult aspects of your life, or simply responding to old stressors more serenely. Either way, your adrenals will thank you—and your life is likely to improve. (To learn more, see http://emdria.org.)

The Work of Byron Katie

When Jenna saw her daughter become frantic about not being able to please her teacher by doing her homework "perfectly," she realized the extent to which her own perfectionism had affected her daughter. Without meaning to, Jenna had somehow modeled for Olivia a lesson of her own childhood, indirectly telling her own daughter what she herself was told: "You need to be perfect in order to be loved and appreciated; if you're not perfect all the time, you will disappoint the people you love."

Many of us have learned this lesson early and all too well. The debilitating sense that "whatever you do, it's not enough" can sap even the most outstanding accomplishment and undermine even the most fulfilling life. Our fears of not being good enough, our need to perpetually compensate for our inadequacies, our compulsion to continually apologize for our shortcomings may seem rational to us, but in fact, these attitudes and behaviors only reveal how much we're still responding to fears of not being able to win our parents' love.

Perfectionism often makes us very judgmental of ourselves and others as we expect too much from ourselves and everybody else. It keeps us from having fun, enjoying our own accomplishments, and fully communicating our love to our children, partners, and friends.

If you feel burdened by excessive self-criticism, judgmentalism, or other aspects of perfectionism, I invite you to explore "The Work" of Byron Katie, a spiritual leader whose process has been praised in *Time* and *O* magazines. Katie suggests identifying every one of your judgmental or self-critical thoughts and then exploring it with the following questions:

- Is it true?

- Can you absolutely know that it's true?

- How do you react, what happens, when you believe that thought?

- Who would you be without that thought?

Then Katie suggests exploring what happens when you turn the thought around. If your thought was "I'm so fat, and that makes me really ugly," you might turn that around to "I'm not fat at all" or "I'm so fat, and that makes me beautiful" or "I really enjoy being fat." The point is not that either thought is false—or true—but rather that neither is the whole truth, and that both have powerful effects on how you see yourself and the world. Becoming aware of your thoughts and their effects, perceiving a truth that is larger than your thoughts, and discovering your power to transform thoughts that seemed unalterably true can all be extremely helpful in liberating you from the perils of perfectionism. (For more information, see www.thework.com.)

Codependent No More

I've taken the title for this section from the groundbreaking book on codependency, *Codependent No More*, by inspirational author Melody Beattie. A struggling single parent working as a freelance writer, Beattie decided in 1986 to write about what happened to people who were involved in relationships with alcoholics or drug addicts. Her concept of codependency has since been expanded to include any of us who see our own identity in terms of others. The classic humorous definition of codependency is that when you're in an accident, *everyone else's* life flashes before your eyes, rather than your own.

I've often thought that women are trained from birth to become codependent, simply because so much of our identity depends on pleasing and taking care of others. If we've grown up believing that "good girls" make *other* people happy, it can seem unutterably selfish to want to make *ourselves* happy, let alone to say no to other people in favor of ourselves.

This was certainly an issue that Jenna struggled with as she sought to care for her husband, children, clients, and friends. What brought home to her the dark side of that behavior was seeing her daughter's nearly hysterical distress. Why, Jenna thought, had Olivia not been able to say *no* to the long line of friends whose calls that evening had kept her from finishing her homework? Why, if Olivia had wanted to prioritize helping friends over completing her work, could she then not say *no* to her teacher's perceived wish that she do a perfect extra-credit assignment? Why had it been so difficult for Olivia to make her own decisions about how she wanted to spend her evening, rather than responding to the demands of one person after another?

If codependency is an issue in your life, you might also begin your exploration of codependency by completing the following exercise:

What Happens When I Say *No?*

Set a timer and commit to writing about one of these questions for at least five continuous minutes. As you write, let go of self-criticism, judgment, and expectation. Simply write as quickly and spontaneously as possible. Even if you think you've run out of ideas, keep writing. Use phrases such as "I don't know what to say now," over and over, until you find yourself moving on.

- What would happen if I said *no* more often?

- Who do I wish I could say *no* to and why?

- What would I do for myself if I woke up one day and had no obligations and total permission to do anything I liked?

- Who would be upset with me if I started saying *no?*

- When was the first time I remember thinking that I shouldn't say *no?*

Once the timer goes off, feel free to keep writing or, if you prefer, take a brisk walk or find some other physical way to blow off the energy that might have built up during this exercise. The next day, write about the experience of answering whichever question you chose and decide how you feel about the experience now.

12-Step Support Groups

An extremely useful way to rewrite the scripts of codependency is to work with a 12-step support group such as Al-Anon (for the loved ones of alcoholics) or ACA (Adult Children of Alcoholics, for those who grew up with alcoholic parents and caretakers). Often, these groups are open to people who appreciate their approach, whether or not their loved ones or caretakers had a physical addiction. Sometimes they help you identify that a parent was, in fact, addicted to a physical substance, even though no one in the family recognized or acknowledged it. Sometimes they help you identify an emotional pattern, such as "rage-aholism," in which angry bursts of temper function much as drunken binges, even if no alcohol is involved. They also identify a pattern known as "being a dry drunk," in which alcoholic behavior continues even when the person is sober. I have been astounded, when I've come to learn more about my patients, at the profound effect an alcoholic or addicted person can have on family life—even two or three generations later. Almost always, these support groups can help you identify—and then rewrite—your own role in the codependent drama, seeing where you participate and helping you find new ways of opting out.

If you think a 12-step support group might be helpful to you, I urge you to locate one online (you might begin at www.12step.org) or in your telephone directory. You might also ask at a local religious or community institution. Most groups have "open meetings" where you're free to check out the process and see if it appeals to you. There can be something almost magical in finding other people who are working on the same issues that you are, committed to rewriting their old responses and replacing them with healthy new ones. With or without traditional "talk therapy" in the background, a 12-step program might help you create new patterns of behavior—and restore your adrenal health.

The Hoffman Process

An extremely powerful healing tool, and one that I myself have engaged in, is the Hoffman Process, an eight-day intensive course that incorporates automatic writing, guided visualizations, and a host of other experiential techniques to help you get in touch with painful childhood experiences and relationships and then to rework your responses to them. If you're willing to explore your deepest feelings about the issues that are holding you back, you may be delighted with the emotional freedom that can result.

Whenever I think about the power of the Hoffman Process, my patient Rebecca comes to mind. In her early 30s, Rebecca had grown a successful business crafting jewelry and, as we talked, she seemed confident and well adjusted. But something changed when Rebecca got up on the exam table. Her shoulders and knees tensed up, and her arms crossed stiffly over her belly. She seemed frightened and defensive as I did her pelvic exam. When she was dressed again, I asked her about it. Rebecca told me she had been having intense pelvic pain for years. As a result, she hadn't been intimate with her husband in months and now he was seeing another woman. I asked if there was anything else going on emotionally, but she simply looked at me and asked, "What does that have to do with my pain?"

Rebecca had done a few years of "talk therapy," where she had learned a great deal about herself. However, like many of us, she had found it all too easy to "talk around" the therapist and convince herself that she could manage on her own. And, like many of us, she had told herself to stop dwelling on her negative feelings because they simply weren't "productive."

Unfortunately, if you don't somehow resolve your negative feelings, they won't simply go away—and they can cause you both emotional and physical pain for years until you work through them. Rebecca had managed to build an extraordinarily successful life. Yet she suffered ongoing intimate pain, and, like Jenna and many of my other patients, showed signs of adrenal dysfunction. The unrelenting stress of keeping the past at bay was taking its toll.

Burying our emotions only means they will resurface some other way, some other time. They may manifest as physical problems or again as unwanted emotional states, but you can be certain that repressed emotions will come back. This was strikingly demonstrated by the Adverse Childhood Experiences (ACE) Study, which found that the more emotional stress people endured as children, the more likely they were to suffer from heart disease, cancer, and other chronic health problems later in life.

What I find so hopeful about the Hoffman Process is the opportunity it offers us to free ourselves from these emotional traps. When we become aware of our feelings—without judgment—simply noticing them and experiencing them—we can begin to put them in perspective. We can move past the overwhelming pain, anger, and helplessness of a child to the wiser and more compassionate view of an adult. We can't skip any steps, however; we have to experience our childhood pain and then release it.

ASK YOURSELF . . .

Can you benefit from further self-exploration? Here are some questions you might ask yourself. If you find yourself answering *yes* to several of them, consider going further with one of the approaches mentioned in this chapter.

- I feel that something is holding me back and want to take the limits off.

- I experience too much stress, and I'm not having enough fun.

- I know what I should do, but often can't generate the will to do it.

- I often feel angry, resentful, embarrassed, or depressed.

- I flip-flop between dominating and intimidating people below me and avoiding being dominated by people above me.

- I feel intimidated, coerced, and manipulated and can't stand up for myself.

- I work compulsively, often to the detriment of other aspects of my life.

- Meaning is going out of my marriage, my career, or life in general. I often feel I'm just going through the motions.

- There's a lack of intimacy in my life—I've been unsuccessful in creating relationships.

- I'm either unemotional or disconnected from my feelings or my feelings are running me.

- I'm in recovery from substance abuse (clean and sober for 90 days minimum) and want to deal with the original pain that led to addiction.

- I recognize that my parents were not as loving and supportive as I wanted them to be, or that bad things happened in my childhood.

- I see myself passing my own suffering on to my children.

Used with the permission of the Hoffman Institute.

Negative Love

One emotion holding many of us back is *negative love:* our tendency to repeat the behaviors we used to win our parents' love; and to repeat our parents' attitudes, behaviors, and treatment of us. If our mother was hypercritical, we might see excessive criticism as an expression of love, and we either become overly critical ourselves or seek out critical people—or both. Likewise, if our father was overly anxious, constantly cautioning us against exploring the world, taking risks, or expressing our true feelings, we too are likely to become anxious and/or surround ourselves with anxious people.

Jenna saw this vividly demonstrated in her daughter's behavior. Just as her mother had taught Jenna to think constantly of how to work harder and please more people, Jenna had inadvertently passed the same lesson on to her daughter. No doubt Jenna's mother had learned this pattern from her mother, who had learned it from *her* mother. Generation after generation passed on the same type of negative love, viewing perfectionism and codependency as precious gifts rather than patterns that hold one back.

If you are interested in exploring the role of negative love in your life, consider trying one or both of the following exercises:

Exploring Negative Love

1. Allow yourself at least 15 minutes for this exercise. Begin with 2 minutes of relaxation through deep breathing—breathing in on a count of 2, then 4, then 6, then 8, then 12, with an exhale of the same length.

2. Identify a behavior you find very hurtful, whether in yourself or others. Set a timer and commit to writing for at least 5 continuous minutes about a recent experience when either you directed that behavior at someone, or someone in your life directed it at you.

3. Reset the timer for another 5 minutes. Now write about a time in your childhood when you experienced this behavior, either in yourself or someone you loved. Choose the first example that comes to mind, and don't worry if, as you write, it morphs into something else.

4. With your remaining time, write about this question: *Now that I have identified this pattern, what would I like to do about it?*

Visualize Love

1. Allow yourself at least 17 minutes for this exercise. Begin with 2 minutes of relaxation through deep breathing—breathing in on a count of 2, then 4, then 6, then 8, then 12, with an exhale of the same length.

2. Set your timer for 5 minutes and picture your parents together at the happiest time you can imagine. It might be a time you actually witnessed or it may be a time you can only imagine: their wedding day, their first date, a tender moment between them. Your goal is to imagine the best version of the love between them, the most positive experience that they could share. Don't force anything; simply allow the images to come to you and notice how they make you feel. If you find yourself unable to imagine any happy moments between your parents, allow yourself to notice how *that* makes you feel.

3. Now set your timer for 5 minutes and picture your parents at one of the worst moments between them—either a moment you actually witnessed or one that you can only imagine. Again, notice what you can about your image, allowing it simply to emerge into your mind's eye and to affect you emotionally however it will.

4. Set your timer for the final 5 minutes, and write without stopping about what you have learned. You can write "freestyle" or attempt to answer the following questions:

   • What did my parents' relationship teach me about love?

   • What do I want to take with me from that lesson?

   • What would I like to do differently from them?

Forgiveness, Healing, and Self-discovery

Over many years of exploring ways to release childhood pain, in my own life and the lives of my patients, I've realized that the key to laying down our emotional burdens is letting go of judgment and embracing forgiveness—of those who hurt us, yes, but also of ourselves. As a medical practitioner, I was delighted to come across the following quote from the co-founder of Harvard University's Mind/Body Clinic, Joan Borysenko, because of the integrative vision blending biochemistry, emotion, and spirit:

> I can tell you as a biologist that when we step into the part of ourselves that doesn't judge, that is simply open to the possibilities of the moment, that what happens is we feel a sense of peace and gratitude. Enormous biochemical changes accompany that, changes in the neuropeptides from the emotional center of the brain, changes in our immune system and our cardiovascular system that are all consistent with good health.

Certainly this was true for Rebecca. As she began to work through her emotional issues, she was able for the first time to explore the sexual abuse she experienced in her early teens from her uncle. Though she'd never forgotten this traumatic experience, she hadn't seen how it had shaped her relationships with everyone from that time forward.

Accepting that painful portion of her past also helped Rebecca recognize a pattern in herself of extreme criticism and judgment, of both herself and others. Just as her family had told her, she would repeat to herself, "You're too sensitive. . . . Lighten up. . . . You're never happy." Knowing that she had had reason to be "sensitive" to her uncle's bad treatment, but choosing now not to keep replaying those harsh words to herself or anyone else, Rebecca slowly but surely began to move forward. For the first time in her life, she felt truly free: from her family's expectations, from the hold her uncle had had on her body, and most of all, from the negative chatter inside her own head. When she got to this quiet place, she told me it was almost scary because she realized, *If I'm not all these things my family has been telling me I am, then who am I?*

And so Rebecca began the work of redefining herself. Although things didn't work out with her husband, she now believes that her marriage ended for the right reasons. And to her delight, she is completely free now of the pelvic pain she'd suffered from for so many years.

As we have seen, Jenna was also able to redefine herself into a more colorful and striking presence, one who modeled joy and self-love for her daughter and her son. For both Jenna and Rebecca, there were four keys: *awareness, release, forgiveness,* and *transformation.* If you would like to further explore these states, consider one or more of the exercises that follow:

1. Awareness

- *Create a stress biography.* When did your stress begin? When did it escalate? What trigger points pushed it higher? Have there ever been any points where it eased up? When and why? Create a time line that identifies your "stress history." Then see what that tells you about what in your life has been working for you and what you might like to change.

- *Basket of burdens/basket of blessings.* What is adding to your allostatic load? Set a timer for 5 minutes and list as many burdens in your basket as you can in that time. If you need more time, keep going. Then set your timer for another 5 minutes and list as many blessings in your life as you can— everything you have to be grateful for, including your ability to read these words and write a list. If specific action occurs to you, go with it, but don't press—your goal at this point is simply to become aware.

2. Release

- *Let it out.* We hold anger and resentment in our physical bodies, so it makes sense that we need to release these emotions in a physical way. Dancing, running, drumming, hitting a pillow with a wiffle-ball bat, or simply letting it out in tears are all ways to physically release your frustration and anger. It's important not to confront the individual who is triggering you while you are highly emotionally activated. In most cases, carrying this anger into a conversation leads us right back to the very pattern we're trying to understand and de-energize.

- *Healing touch.* Sometimes we need support to release powerful emotions. Consider using one of the modalities described in this chapter and the previous one—especially massage, Feldenkrais, polarity therapy, and any other approach that involves being touched—to help you release and unblock.

3. Forgiveness: From Child to Child

The concept for this exercise was taken from the Hoffman Process.

1. Allow yourself at least 30 minutes for this exercise. Begin with 2 minutes of relaxation through deep breathing—breathing in on a count of 2, then 4, then 6, then 8, then 12, with an exhale of the same length.

2. Sit quietly and imagine one of your parents as a child—the one with whom you feel you have the most troubled relationship. Allow the image simply to come into your mind. What age are you imagining? What is the expression on the child's face? Is the child active or sitting quietly or perhaps fidgeting or worrying or even crying? Notice your own reactions as well. How do you feel as you observe this child?

3. Now imagine yourself as a child. Again, allow the image simply to come into your mind, simply observing as details emerge: age, facial expression, activity, and anything else you notice. Notice as well your own reactions to seeing yourself as a child. What is your impulse toward that child? Do you feel angry, protective, sad, proud, fearful? Without judging, simply allow your observations and emotions to be present.

4. When you are ready, begin to write a letter from the part of yourself that is still a child to the part of your parent that is a child. Ask your parent's child about the behavior of your parent that most troubles you. Invite your parent's child to explain why he or she behaves that way and how he or she feels about it.

5. When you are ready, write the reply, as you imagine your parent's child might do. How would he or she answer your questions?

6. After you have finished writing your parent's reply, thank your parent's child for sharing this personal information with you. You may do this in writing or by speaking aloud, but I encourage you to externalize your response—don't simply think it or hear it inside your own head. Express any other feelings you would like to share with your parent's child, including anger, sorrow, fear, or joy. In your mind's ear, hear that other child's response and allow him or her to leave.

7. By yourself, as an adult, write for up to 5 minutes, expressing your thoughts and feelings about what just happened. If possible, revisit your journal every few days for the next couple of weeks, continuing to explore the experience—or repeat the exercise with either the same or the other parent until you feel you have gotten what you needed from the communication.

4. Transformation: Practicing the New

1. Ask a trusted friend or sibling the following question: What have I adopted from my parents that might not be serving me well in my life? Or, more simply: How am I like Mom and Dad—the bad as well as the good? Encourage the other person to speak for a few minutes with no interruptions as you listen carefully and take notes. Focus on listening without judgment, simply to absorb the information.

2. Whether or not you agree, thank your loved one for answering your question. Then allow yourself at least ten minutes every other day for a week to write in your journal about how you feel. Is there some truth to what you heard? A lot of truth? No truth? Why do you think you adopted that behavior? Would you like to give it up? With what would you like to replace it?

3. When you are ready, promise yourself to notice every time you engage in the behavior you would like to change. Begin simply by noticing.

4. When you are ready, follow up your noticing by altering your behavior. If you can alter it before the fact, that's terrific. If you don't catch yourself in time, apologize and do it over again. For example, if you would like to replace excessive criticism with setting a clear boundary plus appreciation, your conversation might go something like this:

    •   *[old way, excessive criticism]:* I don't see why you always have to be late for every one of our meetings!

    •   *[catching yourself and apologizing]:* Wait, I'm sorry, I was being very critical just now.

- *[expressing a clear boundary plus appreciation]:* I really love it when you're on time, and it's so much easier for me when you are.

Continue to practice replacing your old, unwanted behavior with a new behavior. It may take a while, but eventually, the new behavior will come to seem more natural than the old.

Supporting Yourself

Throughout most of this chapter, we've focused on ways you can begin to alleviate stress and heal your adrenal dysfunction by rewriting your responses to childhood pain. This type of emotional work can be challenging, scary, and sometimes painful in its own right. It's all the more important, then, to find as many ways as you can to support yourself. Here are some suggestions for how to do that:

- *List things that make you feel great.* Jot down all the things you can do to make yourself feel wonderful: eat well, get your body moving, surround yourself with loving people, and so on. What else can you think of? Start by making the list—then see if you can manage just one thing a week . . . then every other day . . . then maybe even once a day.

- *Check your support system.* Often, as we start building our self-esteem and understanding the patterns that don't work for us, we begin to realize that we've included people in our circle of intimates who replicate the conflicts and hurtful experiences we had with our parents. Then, as we become healthier and more self-loving, we start becoming less attracted to these repeat instances of "negative love." Consider doing an inventory of your support system—the people you see and speak to frequently and by choice, including family members, friends, and your romantic partner or spouse. Ask yourself how you feel about yourself and your life after spending time with each one. Perhaps you'll realize that spending time with Jane leaves you feeling confused or anxious, whereas talking to Mary always perks you up or calms you down. Consider, then, how to surround yourself only with people who help you create *positive* loving relationships and leave the negative love behind.

A wise and cherished colleague once told me, "You know why we're all so good at using negative patterns? Because we've been practicing them since early childhood." It's so true. And we can take comfort in the fact that health-defeating interactions with others are learned behaviors, behaviors that we can unlearn with time and practice. The best part is that when we release these patterns and come from a place of love emotionally, it can trigger healing physically in the body. That's what Rebecca, Jenna, and thousands of my patients have found. If you are willing to become aware, release your past, forgive yourself and those who have hurt you, and move on to a new action, that healing is there for you, too.

CONCLUSION

LIFE WITHOUT ADRENAL DYSFUNCTION

If you are struggling with adrenal dysfunction, the challenges can seem daunting. You wonder what is wrong with you, why you're so wired and tired, why you've gained weight, why you feel so discouraged. You wonder why no medical practitioner seems able to help you, why no diet seems to work, why the exercise that once made you feel fabulous now leaves you feeling exhausted and drained.

I know how difficult this condition can be. But I'm here to tell you not to give up, because there is hope on the horizon.

First, while medical opinion has been slow to recognize adrenal dysfunction, I do believe that within 25 years, adrenal dysfunction will become a completely accepted diagnosis and that it will be "standard of care" for physicians and practitioners of all types to properly test for it and treat it. The science—in such prestigious publications as the *New England Journal of Medicine, Psychoneuroimmunology,* and *Neuroscience & Biobehavioral Reviews*—is absolutely there. But as we've seen with many other conditions, standard medical practice often takes quite some time to catch up with cutting-edge research. (If you're interested in reading more about the scientific foundation for this book, check out the Further Reading section. For complete documentation, see my websites, www.MarcellePick.com and www.womentowomen.com.)

I don't blame the practitioners. I understand how busy they are and how easily they can become overwhelmed by the plethora of scientific studies that grow more numerous every year. But some of those same studies have demonstrated that it takes standard medical practice at least 50 years to catch up with research findings—and we've only had the data on adrenal dysfunction for just about 25 years. Here's hoping that 25 years from now, this book will have become obsolete—because you've learned everything in these pages from your own medical practitioner!

Meanwhile, I think there are more immediate reasons to be hopeful for every woman who is reading this book. I find it tremendously exciting to know that neither genetics nor our families determine our destiny—that whatever physical traits or emotional baggage we initially inherited from our parents, we have a great deal of power to transform our bodies, minds, and spirits in the direction that we choose. I find it reassuring that how we feel today is not necessarily how we are going to feel tomorrow—the fatigue, weight gain, and emotional issues that plague us are absolutely changeable if we only have the right tools. I've seen so many thousands of women come into my office feeling exhausted, bewildered, and in despair—and I've seen so many thousands recover their energy, their well-being, and their joy.

Many of us have been told—by our practitioners, families, or society itself—that we are too old to change; or that weight gain, exhaustion, and a loss of energy are the inevitable companions of aging. But both the research I have reviewed and the patients I have treated offer ample evidence that this is simply not true. You're never too old to change. You're never too old to lose weight, regain your energy, and face life with a sense of wonder and delight. You may be able to make several changes quickly, or you may need to dig in for a long haul. Either way, if you are determined to make things better for yourself, you absolutely can.

It's true that we are facing new challenges these days, not the least of which are the burdens placed on us by an increasingly toxic environment. Mercury in our fish, PCBs in our water, parabens in our shampoo, and bysphenol in our kitchens add up to increasing levels of heavy metals, xenoestrogens, and other toxic invaders in our bodies. Our nonstop schedules and erratic economy only add to the stress. But we also have new resources to deal with these challenges, including the suggestions and solutions that I share with you in this book.

The ultimate challenge, I think, is to not give up hope, so that we have the wherewithal to make the changes that will improve our lives. Certainly, that's what Tanya—and Katie and Madison and thousands of my other patients—found. Once they made the dietary and lifestyle changes we discussed and started taking the nutritional supplements, they discovered new reserves of physical and emotional energy, enabling them to undertake the emotional work with clarity and commitment. When Tanya came into my office a month after her initial visit, she almost glowed with a quiet sense of serenity and inner purpose. "I'm sleeping way better," she told me, "and I went out twice after work last week! I'm concentrating better, too, getting more done in less time. I'm way less irritable, and way more energized. It's such a relief." She flashed me one of her dazzling smiles, then, suddenly, grew serious. "You know the best thing, though?" she told me. "For the first time in a long, long time, I finally feel like myself."

What better goal for any of us—to feel like the best version of ourselves? As you continue on your journey toward health and well-being, that is my hope and my wish for you.

APPENDIX A

ADDISON'S DISEASE AND CUSHING'S SYNDROME

These conditions are fairly rare. If you have either Addison's disease or Cushing's syndrome, you're likely to receive a different type of treatment than I have suggested in this book. However, the majority of women I treat do *not* have either Addison's or Cushing's and are able to benefit from the 30-day Solution to Adrenal Dysfunction.

Addison's disease is a kind of extreme adrenal insufficiency characterized by chronic fatigue, muscle weakness, loss of appetite, and, usually, weight loss. Other symptoms can include nausea, vomiting, diarrhea, a craving for salty foods, hypoglycemia (low blood sugar), headache, sweating, irregular or absent menstrual periods, and low blood pressure that falls further upon standing, which may cause dizziness or fainting. Sometimes the skin can darken, especially on the lips, skin folds, pressure points (elbows, knuckles, knees, and toes), and mucous membranes, such as the lining of the cheek. Scars may also darken.

A progressive disease, Addison's may resemble other conditions until a stress to the system, such as an illness or accident, causes symptoms to become more severe. In these cases, a person might experience severe vomiting and diarrhea; dehydration; sudden penetrating pain in the lower back, abdomen, or legs; low blood pressure; or loss of consciousness. An Addisonian crisis can even be fatal if not treated.

In less severe types of adrenal dysfunction, the adrenal glands are underperforming but they remain intact. In Addison's, however, the adrenals have been partially destroyed. In about 80 percent of Addison's disease cases, an autoimmune disorder has caused the gradual destruction of the *adrenal cortex,* the adrenal glands' outer layer, which has been attacked by antibodies produced by the immune system.

In other cases, Addison's results from tuberculosis, an infection that destroys the adrenal glands. Addison's disease may also have been caused by chronic infection, particularly fungal infections; AIDS-associated infections; cancer spreading from other parts of the body into the adrenal glands; bleeding into the adrenal glands; *amyloidosis,* a disease that causes abnormal protein buildup in various organs; and various types of genetic defects.

Addison's disease is initially diagnosed with two tests to determine cortisol levels. The ACTH stimulation test measures cortical levels in the blood and/or urine before and after a synthetic form of ACTH is administered. As we saw in Chapter 1, ACTH is the abbreviation for *adrenocorticotropic hormone,* the biochemical that stimulates the adrenals. When the adrenals are functioning normally, an ACTH injection causes a rise in cortisol levels. People with Addison's disease and some other forms of adrenal insufficiency show little or no response to the ACTH.

Another exam, the CRH stimulation test, can reveal more about the causes of adrenal problems. CRH—*corticotropin-releasing-hormone*—is the biochemical that the hypothalamus uses to set off the stress response. Synthetic CRH may be injected so that a person's blood-cortisol levels can be measured 30, 60, 90, and 120 minutes after the injection and compared with a baseline measurement taken previously. Those with Addison's disease respond to a CRH injection by producing high levels of ACTH but no cortisol. An absent ACTH response suggests that the pituitary is causing the adrenal problems, while a delayed ACTH response indicates that the hypothalamus may be at the root of the condition.

If Addison's disease has been diagnosed, blood tests may be ordered to detect the antibodies that would indicate an autoimmune condition. Possibly, an X-ray or ultrasound will be ordered to check for calcium deposits in the adrenals, suggesting adrenal bleeding or, perhaps, tuberculosis, which may also be diagnosed through a skin test. Doctors may order additional tests to explore the condition of the pituitary.

Addison's disease may be treated by prescribing synthetic glucocorticoids to replace the cortisol that the body is not making naturally. Hydrocortisone, prednisone, or dexamethasone may be prescribed, perhaps along with fludrocortisone acetate to treat the aldosterone deficiency that can also result from Addison's.

Addison's disease results from insufficient cortisol. On the other hand, *Cushing's syndrome,* or hypercortisolism, is a hormonal disorder resulting from the body's exposure to excess cortisol. Risk factors for Cushing's syndrome include obesity, type 2 diabetes, fluctuating blood-sugar levels, and high blood pressure.

Symptoms vary, but generally include severe fatigue, muscle weakness, high blood pressure, high levels of blood sugar, increased thirst and urination, and a fatty hump between the shoulders. People with Cushing's typically have upper body obesity, fat around the neck, and rounded faces, along with relatively slender arms and legs. Their skin may become thin and fragile so that it bruises easily and heals slowly. Pink or purple stretch marks may be seen on the arms, breasts, abdomen, thighs, and buttocks. Cushing's syndrome weakens the bones so that bending, lifting, or even standing up may cause backaches or fractures of the ribs or spinal column. Women may develop excess hair on their face, neck, chest, abdomen, and thighs, along with irregular or absent menstrual periods. Men may experience low sex drive, erectile dysfunction, and decreased fertility. People with Cushing's may also suffer from irritability, anxiety, or depression.

The exposure to excess cortisol that results in Cushing's syndrome may have a variety of causes. Some 70 percent of Cushing's syndrome cases result from *adenomas,* small, benign tumors that cause the pituitary to secrete excess ACTH. Sometimes the condition results from consumption of glucocorticoids—steroid hormones that resemble the body's own cortisol. This type of medication is often prescribed in the form of prednisone for asthma, rheumatoid arthritis, lupus, and other inflammatory diseases; or given to suppress immune function to keep the body from rejecting a newly transplanted organ. *Ectopic ACTH syndrome* results from benign or cancerous tumors that arise outside the pituitary and produce their own ACTH. Very rarely, an adrenal tumor or other adrenal abnormality causes the condition.

Cushing's syndrome is diagnosed through a variety of tests, including X-rays of the adrenal and pituitary glands, which may help to locate tumors. Three other lab tests may help practitioners diagnose Cushing's syndrome:

- *24-hour urinary cortisol level.* Urine samples taken several times during a 24-hour cycle are tested for cortisol, with excessively high cortisol levels indicating the possibility of Cushing's.

- *Midnight plasma cortisol and late-night salivary cortisol measurements.* Since cortisol levels are normally far lower at night, midnight blood tests or late-night saliva tests can help determine whether a person has Cushing's syndrome. The test is generally conducted during a 48-hour hospital stay to make sure that stress hasn't caused falsely elevated cortisol levels, though sometimes samples can be taken at home.

- *Low-dose dexamethasone suppression test (LDDST).* The LDDST test usually involves administering a low dose of *dexamethasone,* a synthetic glucocorticoid, every six hours for two days, though in some cases, patients are given only a onetime overnight dose. Urine samples are taken before the dexamethasone is given and then several times thereafter. In a healthy body, dexamethasone causes a drop in blood and urine cortisol levels, so if cortisol remains high, Cushing's syndrome may be the cause. However, various conditions can interfere with the test, which may not cause cortisol to drop in people suffering from depression, alcoholism, high estrogen levels, acute illness, or stress, incorrectly indicating that the person has Cushing's syndrome. Drugs such as phenytoin and phenobarbital may cause cortisol levels to drop, incorrectly suggesting that someone does *not* have Cushing's syndrome.

- *Dexamethasone/corticotropin-releasing hormone (DEX/CRH) test.* Some people have high cortisol levels resulting from depression or anxiety disorders, excess alcohol consumption, poorly controlled diabetes, or severe obesity. However, they don't suffer from the other symptoms of Cushing's. The DEX/CRH test distinguishes pseudo-Cushing's from actual Cushing's: the patient is given dexamethasone and then a CRH stimulation test. In a person without Cushing's, the dexamethasone will prevent the CRH injection from secreting excess cortisol, whereas those with Cushing's syndrome will continue to produce high levels of the hormone.

If Cushing's syndrome is diagnosed, practitioners may order additional tests to help locate the abnormality that is causing high cortisol production. Treatment for Cushing's varies depending upon the reasons for the excess cortisol. Options include surgery, radiation, chemotherapy, and medications that inhibit cortisol.

APPENDIX B

ALLOSTATIC LOAD

To find out your allostatic load, or to get more information about what an allostatic load is, check out the following websites:

- www.allostatix.com

- www.macses.ucsf.edu/research/allostatic/allostatic.php

- www.dana.org/news/publications/detail.aspx?id=4338

- http://stresseraser.com/allostatic-load/

- http://allostaticoverload.com

- http://nursing.unc.edu/bbl/abstracts/logan_barksdale_2008.pdf

APPENDIX C

GLYCEMIC INDEX (GI) AND GLYCEMIC LOAD (GL)

Erratic blood-sugar levels can stress your adrenals, so food choices can make a big difference in recovering from adrenal dysfunction. You ideally want slow, steady support for your blood sugar, rather than foods that will cause your levels to spike and then crash.

Foods with a low glycemic load are most likely to help you achieve stable blood-sugar levels. So when you're choosing what to eat, select more foods with a low glycemic load and fewer with a high glycemic load.

Some discussions of food choices focus on glycemic index, so I have included that number here. But you really don't have to pay too much attention to it. The glycemic index only tells you how much of a rise in blood sugar a certain carbohydrate will produce—not how quickly or slowly your body is likely to metabolize it. The glycemic load is a far more reliable indicator of how a food will affect your blood sugar, and that's the number you should look at, because it indicates the speed at which a carbohydrate will turn into sugar.

Food	GI	Serving Size	Carbs per Serving (g)	GL
Fruits and Juices				
Apple	55	1 medium	21	12
Apricot	57	1 medium	9	5
Banana	51	1 medium	25	13
Carrots, raw	131	½ cup	4	5
Cherries	40	½ cup	12	3
Cranberry juice	105	4 ounces	18	19
Dates, dried	103	2 ounces	40	42
Orange, raw	42	1 medium	11	5
Orange juice	75	6 ounces	20	15
Mango	55	1 cup	17	8
Peach	55	1 medium	11	5
Pear	38	1 medium	11	4
Cereals and Grains				
Bran	72	½ cup	24	17
Cornflakes	81	1 cup	26	21
Oatmeal	82	1 cup	25	21
Raisin bran	88	1 cup	47	41
Rice, brown, boiled	102	1 cup	45	45
Rice, white, boiled	55	1 cup	33	18
Spaghetti, white	58	1½ cups	48	28
Spaghetti, whole wheat	40	1½ cups	42	16
Vegetables				
Russet potato, baked	76	1 medium	30	23
Snack Foods				
Corn chips	46	½ cup	25	11
Doughnut	76	1 medium	23	17
Puffed rice cakes	52	2 cakes	14	12
Bread				
English muffin	86	1 muffin	26	23
Gluten-free multigrain	76	1 slice	13	9

Food	GI	Serving Size	Carbs per Serving (g)	GL
Rye, pumpernickel	41	1 large slice	12	5
White	100	1 large slice	12	12
Whole wheat	60	1 slice	14	8
Dairy and Other				
Skim milk	32	8 ounces	13	4
Soy milk	50	8 ounces	17	8
Yogurt, 2%	40	1 cup	9	3
Legumes and Nuts				
Baked beans	56	1 cup	15	7
Cashews	22	1 ounce	9	2
Chickpeas	32	1 cup	30	3
Kidney beans, dried or boiled	28	1 cup	25	7
Lentils, dried or boiled	29	1 cup	18	5
Peanuts	14	1 ounce	6	1

Adapted from the International Table of Glycemic Index and Glycemic Load Values: 2002 from *The American Journal of Clinical Nutrition* 76 (2002):5–56. Copyright 2002 American Society for Clinical Nutrition. Used by permission.

RESOURCES

Clinical Laboratories

I rely on the following clinical laboratories for much of my diagnostic testing. Their websites offer valuable detailed information about the tests they provide, as well as additional references. Your health-care provider can also use this page as a resource. If you're finding it difficult to get a specific test, you may be able to go through the labs to find a practitioner in your area with whom they've worked before.

Aeron LifeCycles Clinical Laboratory
1933 Davis Street, Suite 310
San Leandro, CA 94577
Phone: 800-631-7900 option 6
www.aeron.com

Aeron LifeCycles offers adrenal testing and a full hormone panel, as well as a non-invasive urine test to determine bone turnover. Evaluated in combination with a bone-density measurement, the rates of bone turnover are used to predict the risk of fracture and the efficacy of treatment therapies. Aeron is one of the few laboratories licensed by the state of New York to accept alternative testing.

Diagnos-Techs, Inc.
19110 66th Avenue South, Building G
Kent, WA 98032
Phone: 800-878-3787
www.diagnostechs.com

Diagnos-Techs also offers adrenal testing and a full hormone panel.

Doctor's Data, Inc.
3755 Illinois Avenue
St. Charles, IL 60174–2420
Phone: 800-323-2784
Phone: 0871-218-0052 (United Kingdom)
Phone: 630-377-8139 (Elsewhere)
www.doctorsdata.com

Doctor's Data, Inc. tests for heavy-metal toxicity, digestive issues, and adrenal function.

Genova Diagnostics
63 Zillicoa Street
Asheville, NC 28801
Phone: 800-522-4762; 828-253-0621
www.genovadiagnostics.com

Genova Diagnostics is a full-service lab that offers a variety of tests, including genetic profiles, adrenal testing, comprehensive parasitology, allergy tests, tests for amino-acid deficiency, stool testing, and tests for liver detoxification (stage one and stage two).

Imugen, Inc.
220 Norwood Park South
Norwood, MA 02062
Phone: 800-246-8436; 781-255-0770
www.imugen.com

Imugen, Inc. tests for tick-borne diseases.

Metametrix Clinical Laboratory
3425 Corporate Way
Duluth, GA 30096
Phone: 800-221-4640; 770-446-5483
www.metametrix.com

Metametrix tests for amino-acid deficiency, allergies, stool and digestive issues, and toxic burden.

NeuroScience, Inc.
373 280th Street
Osceola, WI 54020
Phone: 888-342-7272; 715-294-2144
www.neurorelief.com

This lab tests neurotransmitter levels, amino acids, adrenal function, hormones, and vitamin D levels.

Parasitology Center, Inc. (PCI)
11445 East Via Linda, #2–419
Scottsdale, AZ, 85259–2638
Phone: 480-767-2522
www.parasitetesting.com

PCI tests for parasites and yeast.

ZRT Laboratory
8605 SW Creekside Place
Beaverton, OR 97008
Phone: 866-600-1636; 503-466-2445
www.zrtlab.com

This lab tests hormonal function, vitamin D levels, and cardiometabolic markers.

Cosmetics, Bath, and Beauty

Listed below are products that don't contain parabens, dyes, lead, or other toxins. It's best to choose fragrance-free products. For more information on personal care products, check out the websites for the Environmental Working Group (www.ewg.org) and The Campaign for Safe Cosmetics (www.safecosmetics.org).

Bathtub and Shower Water Filters

- Bathtub and shower head filters (www.santeforhealth.com)

- Crystal Quest Luxury Shower Power filter (http://www.purewaterforless.com/site/675488/product/LSP-WH)

- PiMag Ultra Shower System (www.nikken.com)

- Sprite All-in-One or Slim-Line shower filter (www.bestfilters.com)

Chemical-Free Feminine Hygiene Products

- GladRags (www.gladrags.com)

- Pandora Pads (http://pandorapads.com)

Face and Body Lotions

- Avalon Organics (www.avalonorganics.com)

- Dr. Hauschka skin care products (www.drhauschka.com)

- Ikove by Florestas (www.ikove.com)

- Jurlique skin care (www.jurlique.com)

- Kiss My Face Vitamin A&E Ultra Moisturizer (www.kissmyface.com)

- Organic body care products (www.terressentials.com)

- Pangea Organics (www.pangeaorganics.com)

- Terralina body lotion and fragrance-free body lotion (www.terralina.com)

Hair Products

- By the Planet (www.bytheplanet.com)

- Intelligent Nutrients (www.intelligentnutrients.com)

- La Bella Maria Naturals hair gelle, hair mist, and mousse (www.labellamaria.com)

- Lotus Brands (www.lotusbrands.com)

- Louise Galvin (www.louisegalvin.com)

- Max Green Alchemy (www.maxgreenalchemy.com)

- Morrocco Method International (https://morroccomethod.com)

- Safe hair dyes: (www.ecocolors.net; www.infinitehealthresources.com; http://sunriselaneproducts.com)

- Suki hair products (www.sukiskincare.com)

Makeup

- Eye shadows and mascaras (www.saffronrouge.com)

- Jane Iredale skin care and makeup (www.janeiredale.com)

- La Bella Donna cosmetics (www.labelladonna.com)

Nail Polishes and Removers

- Acquarella chemical-free nail polish (www.ulcw.com)

- Butter London (www.butterlondon.com)

- Honeybee Gardens (www.honeybeegardens.com)

- No-Miss Nail Care (www.nomiss.com)

- Nubar non-carcinogenic nail polish (www.bynubar.com)

- SunCoat Products (www.suncoatproducts.com)

- Zoya (www.zoya.com)

Sunless Tanners

- He-Shi Express Liquid Tan (www.he-shi.com)

- Kiss My Face Instant Sunless Tanner (www.kissmyface.com)

- Lavera Naturkosmetik (www.lavera.com)

Sunscreens

- BADGER SPF 15 for Face and Body (www.badgerbalm.com)

- Burt's Bees Chemical-Free Sunscreeen, SPF 15 and SPF 30 (www.burtsbees.com)

- Erbaviva Sunscreen SPF 15 (www.saffronrouge.com)

- Kiss My Face Sunscreen, SPF 30 and SPF 18, with Oat Protein Complex (www.kissmyface.com)

- Soléo Organics Sunscreen (www.soleoorganics.com)

Exercise and Healing Products

- EmWave Personal Stress Reliever (www.heartmathstore.com/category/emwaveworks)

- X-iser (www.xiser.com)

Light Therapy

- BioBrite, Inc. (www.biobrite.com)

- The SunBox Company (www.sunbox.com)

Food

Gluten-Free Products

You can obtain gluten-free foods from the following sources:

Abigail's Bakery
352 Sugar Hill Road
Weare, NH 03281
Phone: 603-724-6544
www.abigailsbakery.com

Against the Grain Gourmet
22 Browne Court, Unit 119
Brattleboro, VT 05301
Phone: 802-258-3838
www.againstthegraingourmet.com

Sami's Bakery
2339 East Busch Boulevard
Tampa, FL 33612
Phone: 877-989-2722; 813-989-2722
www.samisbakery.com

For more information on gluten and gluten-free products, check out the following websites:

- www.gicare.com/diets/gluten-free.aspx

- http://glutenfreeworks.com/gluten-disorders/gluten/

- www.wisegeek.com/what-is-gluten.htm

A number of gluten-free foods are available. I've listed some brands and products that I have personally used. You can find these and other brands at a health-food store or by ordering online at www.glutenfree.com or www.glutenfreemall.com. Be mindful, though, that just because a product is gluten-free does not ensure that all of its ingredients are healthy and safe for you, so check the labels carefully.

Bagels and Breads

- Abigail's Bakery rolls, breads, and baguettes

- Against the Grain Gourmet sesame bagels

- Better Bread pizza

- Enjoy Life bagels

- Food for Life raisin-pecan bread and brown-rice tortillas

- Glutino frozen bagels, breadsticks (pizza and sesame), biscuits, and original crackers

- Le Garden Bakery bread and croutons

- Sami's Bakery brown-rice and white-rice tortillas

Cereal

- Bakery on Main apple-raisin-walnut granola

- Cream Hill Estates Lara's Rolled Oats

- Nature's Path Mesa Sunrise Flakes

Condiments

- Barkat vegetable-gravy mix

- Esparrago asparagus guacamole

- Hempzels horseradish hemp and honey mustard

- J & S No Nuts Golden Gluten-Free peabutter

- Maxwell's Kitchen chicken-gravy mix

- Mr. Spice Indian curry sauce

Desserts

- Arico chocolate-chip-cookie bar

- Barkat ice-cream cones

- Candy Tree black-licorice vines

- Envirokidz cookies

- Glutino sandwich cookies and chocolate-chip cookies

Entrées

- Amy's frozen entrées

- Chebe frozen pizza

- Foods By George pizza

- Gillian's frozen pizza

- Glutino frozen pizza

Grains

- Shiloh Farms brown basmati rice

- Shiloh Farms kasha

- Shiloh Farms millet grain

Mixes

- Authentic Foods chocolate-cake mix

- Authentic Foods pancake mix

- Betty Crocker gluten-free chocolate-brownie mix

- 'Cause You're Special! cake mix

- 'Cause You're Special! classic sugar-cookie mix

- The Cravings Place all-purpose pancake and waffle mix

- Namaste baking mixes

- Pamela's Products baking and pancake mix

Pasta

- Ancient Harvest quinoa linguine

- Ancient Harvest quinoa pasta elbows

- Glutino macaroni

- Tinkyada brown-rice pasta (all shapes)

- Tinkyada organic brown-rice pasta (all shapes)

- Tinkyada spinach brown-rice spaghetti

- Tinkyada vegetable brown-rice spirals

Snacks

- Barkat sesame pretzels

- Blue Diamond Nut Thins crackers in a wide variety of flavors

- Envirokidz rice bars

- Glutino pretzels and cheddar crackers

- Mary's Gone Crackers (all flavors)

- Schär table crackers

- Trader Joe's onion and chive-seeded corn crackers

Soups

- Celefibr vegetable-bouillon cubes

- Full Flavor Foods chicken-soup stock mix

Yeast-Free Flour

- Bob's Red Mill gluten-free flour

GMO-Free Foods

"GMO" means "genetically modified organism," referring to plants that have been genetically modified to enhance desired traits, such as increased resistance to herbicides or drought; to have higher yields; or to have improved nutritional content. Many scientists and writers have raised concerns about genetically modified foods with regard to environmental hazards, human health risks, and economic concerns. I personally recommend avoiding genetically modified foods if possible, so I'm letting you know that Whole Foods has committed to sourcing all of the ingredients for its store brands from GMO-free sources, and I'm providing you the following list of companies that offer GMO-free products.

Baking Mixes, Flours, Bread, Baked Goods

- Arrowhead Mills

- Bob's Red Mill

- French Meadow Bakery

- Grindstone Bakery

- Pamela's Products

- To Your Health Sprouted Flour Co.

Dairy

- Brown Cow plain yogurt

- FAGE yogurt

- The Greek Gods yogurt

- Pure Indian Foods ghee

- Stonyfield Farm yogurt

Meats, Vegetables

- US Wellness Meats

- Wisconsin Healthy Grown potatoes

Prepared Foods (Soups, Canned Goods, Soy Sauce, Frozen Entrées)

- Amy's Kitchen

- Annie's Naturals

- Cascadian Farm

- Eden Foods

- Genisoy

- Imagine Foods

- Lundberg Family Farms

- Muir Glen

- Natural Choice Foods

- Purity Foods

- San-J

- Spectrum Organic Products

- Thai Kitchen

- Tradition Miso

- Vitasoy

- WhiteWave

- Whole Foods Market products

Snacks, Salsas, Chips, Desserts

- Barbara's Bakery

- Bearitos

- Clif Bar

- Garden of Eatin'

- Kettle Brand chips

- Nature's Path

- Purity Foods

- Que Pasa

- Zukay Live Foods

Household Products

Below is a list of my favorite nontoxic kitchen, bed, and bath products. I have tried to find you products that are attractive, durable, and easy to find at your local health-food store or on the Internet. I use these products at my clinic and in my home, and to the best of my knowledge they are as green as they claim to be. You can also search for products in the Gaiam catalog (www.gaiam.com) and the Whole Earth catalog (www.wholeearth.com), both of which are great resources for nontoxic—or at least, less toxic—home products.

Cleaning Products

Fruit and Vegetable Washes

- Biokleen produce wash (http://biokleenhome.com)

- Environné fruit and vegetable wash

- Fit fruit and vegetable wash

- Womentowomen.com recipe: Put ¼ cup vinegar and 2 tablespoons of salt into a sink or tub of water and let your vegetables and fruits soak for 15 minutes. You can add baking soda to scrub fruits as well. Be sure to rinse thoroughly after soaking.

Heat and Therapy Packs

- Grampa's Garden vapo heat pillow (www.grampasgarden.com)

Household Cleaning Products

- Citrus Magic (www.citrusmagic.com)

- Earth-friendly products (www.ecos.com)

- Earth's Best laundry detergent, baby wipes, and nursery wipes (www.earthsbest.com)

- Environmentally safe, energy-efficient products (www.greenstore.com)

- Green Feet (www.greenfeet.com)

- Greener Country (www.greenercountry.com)

- Healthy Cleaning (www.healthycleaning.com)

- Mrs. Meyer's Clean Day (www.mrsmeyers.com)

- Sunrise Lane (www.sunriselaneproducts.com)

How to Make Your Own Nontoxic Cleaners

- (www.ehow.com/how_2044781_make-nontoxic-bathroom-cleaners)

Mold

- To remove mold that won't disappear with a good dosing of tea-tree oil: (www.moldadvisor.com)

- For more on how to make your own household products, see *Better Basics for the Home* by Annie Berthold-Bond.

Household and Bedroom Products

Air Filters

- Air Wellness Power5 Pro and Air Wellness Traveler (www.nikken.com)

- Austin Air HealthMate Plus and Austin Air HealthMate Jr. (www.healthpurifiers.com)

- Nordic Pure air filters (www.airfiltershome.com)

- Real Goods air filters and purifiers (www.realgoods.com)

Allergy Relief Products

- Allergy-free bedding and asthma treatments (www.allergyasthmatech.com)

- Allergy-proof mattress and pillow covers (www.allergystore.com)

- Dust-mite mattress and pillow covers (www.allergysolution.com)

- HEPA air filters, dehumidifiers, water filters (www.allergybuyersclub.com)

Home, Housekeeping, and Pest Control

- Green Home environmental store (www.greenhome.com)

Kitchenware

Blenders

- Vitamix blender (www.vitamix.com)

Glass Storage Containers

- Anchor Hocking glass refrigerator storage containers (www.cooking.com)

- Crate and Barrel rectangular glass storage containers (www.crateandbarrel.com)

- Frigoverre glass storage containers with lids (www.chefscatalog.com)

- Pyrex round and rectangle storage containers (www.pyrex.com)

- Snapware glass lock round storage containers (www.bedbathandbeyond.com)

- Williams-Sonoma glass storage containers (www.williams-sonoma.com)

Non-Leaching Baking Pans

- Cabela's cast-iron skillet (www.cabelas.com)

- New Era waterless cookware (www.neweracookware.com)

- Pyrex glass baking pans (www.pyrex.com)

- Tramontina stainless-steel baking/roasting pan (www.qvc.com)

Rice Cookers, Pressure Cookers

- Aeternum pressure cooker (www.healthclassics.com)

- Iwachu Gohan Nabe iron rice cooker (www.zensuke.com)

- Miracle stainless-steel rice cooker (www.ultimate-weight-products.com)

- Small ceramic rice crock (www.kushistore.com)

Tap Water or Drinking Water Filters

- Aquasana healthy-water products (www.aquasana.com)

- K5 Drinking water station (www.kinetico.com)

- PiMag Agua Pour or Pour Deluxe (www.nikken.com)

- PiMag deluxe countertop, or deluxe under-counter water system (www.nikken.com)

- Water filters (www.custompure.com)

Tea Kettles and Teapots

- Ceramic or glass tea kettles (www.theteacorner.com)

- KitchenAid porcelain tea kettle with stainless-steel interior (www.bedbathandbeyond.com)

Vegetable Steamers

- Stainless-steel vegetable steamer (www.norpro.com)

- Stainless-steel vegetable steamer with feet (www.crateandbarrel.com)

- Welco three-piece stainless-steel steamer (www.target.com)

Pest Control

- Bye, Bye Black Fly and No, No Mosquito (http://bearmountainbotanicals.com)

- Nontoxic pest control (http://sunriselaneproducts.com)

Pet Products

- Nontoxic pet products (http://sunriselaneproducts.com)

Medical Therapies

Biodentistry

Many chronic health problems may have been caused by damage from the mercury in dental fillings, root canals, and untreated tooth decay. Biological dentists are trained to recognize the close connection between dental health and body structure, immune and nervous systems, and nutrition. Biological dentists have also been trained to safely remove dental fillings that may contain mercury and replace them with safer materials.

For more information, please read the newsletter furnished by Hal Huggins at Huggins Applied Healing:

Huggins Applied Healing
5082 List Drive
Colorado Springs, CO 80919
Phone: 866-948-4638
www.hugginsappliedhealing.com

To find a practitioner near you, contact:

Foundation for Toxic-Free Dentistry
PO Box 608010
Orlando, FL 32860–8010

Mercury Free Dentists
439 East Thompson
PO Box 154
Amity, AR 71921
Phone: 870-576-9635
www.mercuryfreedentists.com

Body-Based Techniques

Following is a list of some popular body-based techniques used by various health-care practitioners. They may be used alone or in combination with other approaches.

Acupuncture: One of the main elements of traditional Chinese medicine, acupuncture is now widely accepted in Western medicine for the treatment of pain, nausea, and other conditions. Insurance companies reimburse for the cost of acupuncture to treat dozens of diagnoses, a sure sign of acceptance in our culture. Studies support acupuncture's effectiveness for many medical issues, including cramps, dysmenorrhea, and menopausal symptoms. For more information, see www.acupuncture.com.

For anyone in New England, I recommend:

Fern Tsao
Acupuncture Associates of Maine
8 Bennett Road
Yarmouth, ME 04096
Phone: 207-846-4433
www.acupunctureassociatesmaine.com

Aromatherapy: Aromatherapy relies on the healing effects of plants via essential oils and other aromatic compounds, which relax our bodies and stimulate various functions, especially our senses. Essential oils can stimulate the brain's emotional centers, activate thermal receptors on the skin, act as natural antibiotics and fungicides, and possibly enhance the immune response in other ways not yet fully understood. For more information, see www.aromatherapy.com and www.aromaweb.com.

Bach Flower Remedies: Bach Flower Remedies is a system of 38 flower-based compounds developed in the 1930s by English physician and homeopath Edward Bach. The remedies are designed to help correct emotional imbalances. "Rescue Remedy" is the best known Flower Essence, helping individuals to decrease stress, anxiety, and panic attacks. For more information or to find a practitioner who uses this approach, see www.bachflower.com.

Chelation Therapy: Chelation therapy is a form of detoxification that has been used within the alternative medical community for many years to treat patients with dangerous levels of lead and other toxins in their system. A synthetic amino acid known as ethylenediaminetetraacetic acid (EDTA) travels through the body to chelate, or bind, heavy metals and minerals, allowing them to be excreted through urination. A National Institute of Health study is currently under way to evaluate the effectiveness of EDTA chelation therapy for the treatment of coronary-artery disease. Chelation therapy is otherwise not well studied, and it continues to remain controversial. For more information, see http://nccam.nih.gov/health/chelation.

Chiropractic: This system of treatment is based on the premise that good health stems from the unimpeded flow of nerve impulses from the brain and spinal cord to other parts of the body. Misaligned vertebrae of the spine, known as subluxations, disrupt this flow and are accordingly adjusted by the chiropractor along with other joints. Many chiropractors use other natural remedies for adjunctive healing and prevention. All 50 states currently have licensing procedures for chiropractic practitioners. For more information, see http://nccam.nih.gov/health/chiropractic.

Herbal Remedies: Herbalists and many other alternative practitioners rely on herbal medicine, which happens to be the basis for many prescription drugs. Herbal remedies can take the form of teas, tinctures, oils, creams, and pills. Many herbs can be poisonous or interact dangerously with prescription drugs, so it is best to use them only under the supervision of a qualified practitioner. For more information, see www.nlm.nih.gov/medlineplus/herbalmedicine.html.

Massage: One of the oldest forms of healing, massage therapy is used alone or in conjunction with a variety of treatments to alleviate stress and soreness, and to increase blood flow to the muscles. Some forms claim to detoxify, while others offer to open blocked energy channels through applying pressure on certain points in the body. Types of massage include reflexology, Rolfing, shiatsu, Swedish massage, and sports massage. For more information, contact:

American Massage Therapy Association
500 Davis Street, Suite 900
Evanston, IL 60201–4695
Phone: 877-905-0577; 847-864-0123
www.amtamassage.org

Functional Medicine

Functional medicine is a comprehensive approach to health care that treats the whole patient first, not the disease. It integrates the best of Western and ancient modalities, with an emphasis on maintaining organ integrity and subtly shifting core physiology through nutrition and lifestyle.

To find a functional medical practitioner near you, contact:

Institute for Functional Medicine
4411 Point Fosdick Drive NW, Suite 305
PO Box 1697
Gig Harbor, WA 98335
Phone: 800-228-0622
www.functionalmedicine.org

Homeopathy

Founded in early 19th-century Europe, homeopathy is a medical discipline based on the ancient "Law of Similars": substances that cause healthy people to develop symptoms will cure those symptoms in a sick person when administered in infinitesimally small doses. (Vaccines operate on a similar principle.) Using serially diluted remedies from natural sources, homeopaths (most of whom are naturopaths) treat and prevent illness using one medicine at a time at the lowest dosage possible to evoke the required response. Licensing requirements vary from state to state, and you will often find acupuncturists, naturopaths, herbalists, osteopaths (D.O.'s) and medical doctors (M.D.'s) who are also licensed homeopaths. To find one, contact:

National Center for Homeopathy
101 South Whiting Street, Suite 16
Alexandria, VA 22304
Phone: 703-548-7790
www.nationalcenterforhomeopathy.org

Naturopathy

Naturopathy is based on the belief that the body is innately capable of recovering from injury and disease, since health is its natural state. Most naturopaths incorporate elements from various alternative methods, including homeopathy, herbal medicines, acupuncture, nutrition therapy, and bodywork. Naturopathy has its roots in ancient medicinal practices but became a separate discipline in Germany in the 19th century. Founded on the precepts of a medical regimen of hydrotherapy, exercise, fresh air, sunlight, and herbal remedies, this system has evolved today to include a wide spectrum of holistic practitioners. To find one in your area, contact:

American Association of Naturopathic Physicians
4435 Wisconsin Avenue NW, Suite 403
Washington, DC 20016
Phone: 866-538-2267; 202-237-8150
www.naturopathic.org

Bastyr University Naturopathic Medicine Graduate Program
14500 Juanita Drive NE
Kenmore, WA 98028–4966
Phone: 425-823-1300
www.bastyr.edu

Sound-Generating and White-Noise Machines

Sound-Generating Machines

- www.lifescapesmusic.com

- www.newearthrecords.com

- www.relax-and-sleep.com/relaxing-music.html

- www.soundsleeping.com

White-Noise Machines

- www.acousticalsurfaces.com/white_noise/white_noise.htm

- www.purewhitenoise.com/p-67-smooth-radio-static.aspx

- www.soundmachinesdirect.com

Supplements

Look for pharmaceutical-grade supplements. Companies such as the following make high-quality products, many of which I recommend to my patients.

Carlson Nutritional Supplements
15 College Drive
Arlington Heights, IL 60004–1985
Phone: 888-234-5656; 847-255-1600
www.carlsonlabs.com

Designs for Health
980 South Street
Suffield, CT 06078
Phone: 800-367-4325
www.designsforhealth.com

Douglas Laboratories
600 Boyce Road
Pittsburgh, PA 15205
Phone: 800-245-4440
www.douglaslabs.com

Emerson Ecologics
7 Commerce Drive
Bedford, NH 03110
Phone: 800-654-4432
https://emersonecologics.com

Integrative Therapeutics, Inc.
825 Challenger Drive
Green Bay, WI 54311
Phone: 800-931-1709
www.integrativeinc.com

Life Extension Foundation
PO Box 407198
Ft. Lauderdale, FL 33340–7198
Phone: 800-678-8989
www.lef.org

Metagenics
100 Avenida La Pata
San Clemente, CA 92673
Phone: 800-692-9400
www.metagenics.com

NeuroScience, Inc.
373 280th Street
Osceola, WI 54020
Phone: 888-342-7272
www.neurorelief.com

Pure Encapsulations
490 Boston Post Road
Sudbury, MA 01776
Phone: 800 753 2277
www.purecaps.com

Standard Process, Inc.
1200 West Royal Lee Drive
Palmyra, WI 53156
Phone: 800-848-5061; 800-558-8740
www.standardprocess.com

Subtle Engergy Solutions Sales Corp.
8152 Southwest Hall Boulevard #103
Beaverton, OR 97008
http://enzymes.subtleenergysolutions.com

T. E. Neesby, Inc.
9909 North Meridian Avenue
Fresno, CA 93720
Phone: 559-433-3110 Thorne Research, Inc.
PO Box 25
Dover, ID 83825
Phone: 800-747-1950; 208-263-1337
www.thorne.com

XYMOGEN
725 South Kirkman Road
Orlando, FL 32811
Phone: 800-647-6100; 407-445-0203
www.xymogen.com

Websites

Meditation

- www.chopra.com/meditation

- www.freemeditations.com

- www.healthjourneys.com

- www.learningmeditation.com

- www.meditationoasis.com

- www.tm.org

Motivation

- www.motivational-depot.com

Music

- www.healingsounds.com

- www.soundfeelings.com

- www.soundstrue.com

Self-Help Publications and Audio Products

- www.hayhouse.com

Visualization

- http://www.crystalsbay.net/creative-visualization-exercises.html

- http://hypknowsis.com/Visualization-Techniques/LV6-Guided-Visualisation-Exercises.php

- http://www.mjbovo.com/VisualizeSpecific.htm

- www.righthealth.com

- www.stevepavlina.com

- www.suite101.com/content/visualization-on-exercises-a101286

- http://visualizationfx.com/

REFERENCES AND FURTHER READING

For your convenience, I've provided you with this abridged list of references. The notations are listed in the order of the related text in each chapter. While this is not a complete list of the sources used in the publication of this book, these are the most directly related. All the science in this book is fully documented, so for those interested in more depth, see the full version of this bibliography at www.MarcellePick.com.

Introduction

S. J. Lupien, et al., "Stress Hormones and Human Memory Function across the Lifespan," *Psychoneuroendocrinology* 30, no. 3 (April 2005):225–242.

S. J. Lupien, et al., "Cortisol Levels During Human Aging Predict Hippocampal Atrophy and Memory Deficits," *Nature Neuroscience* 1, no. 1 (May 1998):69–73.

M. A. Demitrack, et al., "Evidence for Impaired Activation of the Hypothalamic-Pituitary-Adrenal Axis in Patients with Chronic Fatigue Syndrome," *Journal of Clinical Endocrinology & Metabolism* 73, no. 6 (December 1991):1224–1234.

Gregory Miller, et al. "Chronic Stress Alters Our Genetic Immune Response," *Biological Psychiatry* (August 15, 2008).

S. J. Lupien, et al., "Child's Stress Hormone Levels Correlate with Mother's Socioeconomic Status and Depressive State," *Biological Psychiatry* 48, no. 10 (November 15, 2000):976–980.

George Chrousos and Tomoshige Kino, "Ikaros Transcription Factors: Flying Between Stress and Inflammation," *Journal of Clinical Investigation* 115, no. 4 (2005):844–848.

H. Murakami, et al., "The Frequency of Type 2 Diabetic Patients Who Meet the Endocrinological Screening Criteria of Subclinical Cushing's Disease," *Endocrine Journal* (January 19, 2010).

Jim Connell contact person for *JAMA and Archive Journals* (718-584-9000), "Adult Offspring of Parents with PTSD Have Lower Cortisol Levels," *Archives of General Psychiatry* 64, no. 9 (2007):1040–1048.

Chapter 1

B. M. Kudielka, J. E, Broderick, and C. Kirschbaum, "Compliance with Saliva Sampling Protocols: Electronic Monitoring Reveals Invalid Cortisol Daytime Profiles in Noncompliant Subjects," *Psychosomatic Medicine* 65 (2003):313–319.

K. Richards, et al., "Use of Complementary and Alternative Therapies to Promote Sleep in Critically Ill Patients," *Critical Care Nursing Clinics of North America* 15, no. 3 (September 2003):329–340.

A. J. Yun, P. Y. Lee, J. D. Doux, "Are We Eating More Than We Think? Illegitimate Signaling and Xenohormesis as Participants in the Pathogenesis of Obesity," *Medical Hypotheses* 67, no. 1 (2006):36–40.

C. F. Gillespie and C. B. Nemeroff, "Hypercortisolemia and Depression," *Psychosomatic Medicine* 67, Supplement 1 (2005):S26–S28.

A. J. Dunn, et al., "HPA Axis Activation and Neurochemical Responses to Bacterial Translocation from the Gastrointestinal Tract," Department of Pharmacology and Therapeutics, Louisiana State University Health Sciences Center, Shreveport, Louisiana.

O. T. Wolf, "Stress and Memory in Humans: Twelve Years of Progress?" *Brain Research* 1293 (October 13, 2009):142–154.

P. Chen, et al., "Depression, Another Autoimmune Disease from the View of Autoantibodies," *Medical Hypotheses* 73, no. 4 (October 2009):508–509.

S. Kern, et al., "Glucose Metabolic Changes in the Prefrontal Cortex Are Associated with HPA Axis Response to a Psychosocial Stressor," *Psychoneuroendocrinology* 33, no. 4 (May 2008):517–529.

J. D. Söderholm and M. H. Perdue, "Stress and the Gastrointestinal Tract. II. Stress and Intestinal Barrier Function," *American Journal of Physiology. Gastrointestinal Liver Physiology* 280, no. 1 (January 2001):G7–G13.

M. ter Wolbeek, et al., "Cortisol and Severe Fatigue: A Longitudinal Study in Adolescent Girls," *Psychoneuroendocrinology* 32, no. 2 (February 2007):171–182.

H. Tarui and A. Nakamura, "Saliva Cortisol: A Good Indicator for Acceleration Stress," *Aviation, Space and Environmental Medicine* 58, no. 6 (June 1987):573–575.

C. Bigert, G. Bluhm, and T. Theorell, "Saliva Cortisol—a New Approach in Noise Research to Study Stress Effects," *International Journal of Hygiene and Environmental Health* 208, no. 3 (2005):227–230.

Chapter 2

T. B. VanItallie, "Stress: A Risk Factor for Serious Illness," *Metabolism* 51, no. 6, Supplement 1 (June 2002):40–45.

S. R. Alt, et al., "Differential Expression of Glucocorticoid Receptor Transcripts in Major Depressive Disorder Is Not Epigenetically Programmed," *Psychoneuroendocrinology*, 35, no. 4 (May 2010):544–556.

P. Karling, et al., "Gastrointestinal Symptoms Are Associated with Hypothalamic-Pituitary-Adrenal Axis Suppression in Healthy Individuals," *Scandinavian Journal of Gastroenterology* 42, no. 11 (November 2007):1294–1301.

K. Holtorf, "Data Study Suggests Cortisol Could Alleviate for Chronic Fatigue Syndrome and Fibromyalgia," *Journal of Chronic Fatigue* (2008).

I. Vermes and A. Beishuizen, "The Hypothalamic-Pituitary-Adrenal Response to Critical Illness," *Best Practice & Research Clinical Endocrinology & Metabolism* 15, no. 4 (December 2001):495–511.

B. S. McEwen, "Sex, Stress and the Hippocampus: Allostasis, Allostatic Load and the Aging Process," *Neurobiology of Aging* 23, no. 5 (September–October 2002):921–939.

C. Tsigos and G. P. Chrousos, "Hypothalamic-Pituitary-Adrenal Axis, Neuroendocrine Factors and Stress," *Journal of Psychosomatic Research* 53, no. 4 (October 2002):865–871.

B. S. McEwen, et al., "The Role of Adrenocorticoids as Modulators of Immune Function in Health and Disease: Neural, Endocrine and Immune Interactions," *Brain Research Reviews* 23, no. 1–2 (February 1997):79–133.

S. J. Lupien, et al., "The Modulatory Effects of Corticosteroids on Cognition: Studies in Young Human Populations," *Psychoneuroendocrinology* 27, no. 3 (April 2002):401–416.

M. Justin Kim and Paul J. Whalen, "The Structural Integrity of an Amygdala-Prefrontal Pathway Predicts Trait Anxiety," *The Journal of Neuroscience* 29, no. 37 (September 16, 2009):11614–11618.

M. B. Solomon, et al., "The Medial Amygdala Modulates Body Weight but Not Neuroendocrine Responses to Chronic Stress," *Journal of Neuroendocrinology* 22, no. 1 (January 2010):13–23.

Chapter 3

D. S. Goldstein, I. J. Kopin, "Evolution of Concepts of Stress," *Stress* (Amsterdam, Netherlands) 10, no. 2 (June 2007):109–120.

R. Grassi-Oliveira, M. Ashy, and L. M. Stein, "Psychobiology of Childhood Maltreatment: Effects of Allostatic Load?" *Revista Brasileira de Psiquiatria* 30, no. 1 (March 2008):60–68.

K. Kario, B. S. McEwen, and T. G. Pickering, "Disasters and the Heart: A Review of the Effects of Earthquake-Induced Stress on Cardiovascular Disease," *Hypertension Research* 26, no. 5 (May 2003):355–367.

B. S. McEwen, "Mood Disorders and Allostatic Load," *Biological Psychiatry* 54, no. 3 (August 1, 2003):200–207.

B. S. McEwen, "Plasticity of the Hippocampus: Adaption to Chronic Stress and Allostatic Load," *Annals of the New York Academy of Sciences* 933 (March 2001):265–277.

H. Raff, "Utility of Salivary Cortisol Measurements in Cushing's Syndrome and Adrenal Insufficiency," *Journal of Clinical Endocrinology and Metabolism* 94, no. 10 (October 2009):3647–3655.

I. Bengtsson, et al., "The Cortisol Awakening Response and the Metabolic Syndrome in a Population-Based Sample of Middle-Aged Men and Women," *Metabolism* 59, no. 7 (July 2010):1012–1019.

Chapter 4

W. G. Moons, N. I. Eisenberger, and S. E. Taylor, "Anger and Fear Responses to Stress Have Different Biological Profiles," *Brain Behavior and Immunity* 24, no. 2 (February 2010):215–219.

N. A. Nicolson and R. van Diest, "Salivary Cortisol Patterns in Vital Exhaustion," *Journal of Psychosomatic Research* 49, no. 5 (2000):335–342.

S. Bellingrath, T. Weigl, and B. M. Kudielka, "Cortisol Dysregulation in School Teachers in Relation to Burnout, Vital Exhaustion, and Effort-Reward-Imbalance," *Biological Psychology* 78, no. 1 (April 2008):104–113.

S. Izawa, et al., "Effect of Hostility on Salivary Cortisol Levels in University Students," *Journal of Psychosomatic Research* 49, no. 5 (November 2000):335–342.

K. Pacák, "Stressor-Specific Activation of the Hypothalamic-Pituitary-Adrenocortical Axis," *Physiological Research* 49 Supplement 1 (2000):S11–S17.

S. E. Sephton, et al., "Diurnal Cortisol Rhythm as a Predictor of Breast Cancer Survival," *Journal of the National Cancer Institute* 92, no. 12 (2000):994–1000.

Chapter 5

E. Bay, et al., "Chronic Stress, Salivary Cortisol Response, Interpersonal Relatedness, and Depression among Community-Dwelling Survivors of Traumatic Brain Injury," *Journal of Neuroscience Nursing* 37, no. 1 (February 2005):4–14.

B. S. McEwen, "Protection and Damage from Acute and Chronic Stress: Allostasis and Allostatic Overload and Relevance to the Pathophysiology of Psychiatric Disorders," *Annals of the New York Academy of Sciences* 1032 (December 2004):1–7.

B. S. McEwen, "Early Life Influences on Life-long Patterns of Behavior and Health," *Mental Retardation and Developmental Disabilities Research Reviews* 9, no. 3 (2003):149–154.

J. D. Bremner, et al., "Elevated CSF Corticotropin-Releasing Factor Concentrations in Posttraumatic Stress Disorder," *American Journal of Psychiatry* 154, no. 5 (May 1997):624–629.

C. O. Ladd, M.J. Owens, C.B. Nemeroff, "Persistent Changes in Corticotropin-Releasing Factor Neuronal Systems Induced by Maternal Deprivation," *Endocrinology* 137, no. 4 (April 1996):1212–1218.

M. Weinstock, "The Long-term Behavioural Consequences of Prenatal Stress," *Neuroscience & Biobehavioral Reviews* 32, no. 6 (August 2008):1073–1086.

A. T. de Bruijn, et al., "Prenatal Maternal Emotional Complaints Are Associated with Cortisol Responses in Toddler and Preschool Aged Girls," *Developmental Psychobiology* 51, no. 7 (November 2009):553–563.

D. B. Chamberlain, "Babies Remember Pain," *Pre- and Peri-natal Psychology Journal* 3, no. 4 (1989):297–310.

A. L. Kozyrskyj, et al., "Continued Exposure to Maternal Distress in Early Life Is Associated with an Increased Risk of Childhood Asthma," *American Journal of Respiratory and Critical Care Medicine* 177, no. 2 (January 15, 2008):142–147.

Chapter 6

P. Björntorp, "Do Stress Reactions Cause Abdominal Obesity and Comorbidities?" *Obesity Review* 2, no. 2 (May 2001):73–86.

G. Gastaldi and J. Ruiz, "Metabolic Dysfunction and Chronic Stress: A New Sight at 'Diabesity' pandemic," *Revue Medicale Suisse* 5, no. 206 (June 3, 2009):1273–1277.

M. Shimazaki and J. L. Martin, "Do Herbal Agents Have a Place in the Treatment of Sleep Problems in Long-Term Care?" *Journal of the American Medical Directors Association* 8, no. 4 (May 2007):248–252.

C. Stevinson and E. Ernst, "Valerian for Insomnia: A Systematic Review of Randomized Clinical Trials," *Sleep Medicine* 1, no. 2 (April 1, 2000):91–99.

J. J. Baskett, et al., "Does Melatonin Improve Sleep in Older People? A Randomised Crossover Trial," *Age and Ageing* 32, no. 2 (March 2003):164–170.

P. J. Houghton, "The Scientific Basis for the Reputed Activity of Valerian," *Journal of Pharmacy and Pharmacology* 51, no. 5 (May 1999):505–512.

M. T. Cantorna and B. D. Mahon, "Mounting Evidence for Vitamin D as an Environmental Factor Affecting Autoimmune Disease Prevalence," *Experimental Biology and Medicine* 229, no. 11 (December 2004):1136–1142.

T. Hamazaki, et al., "Anti-stress Effects of DHA," *Biofactors* 13, no. 1–4 (2000):41–45.

L. Bu, K. D. Setchell, and E. D. Lephart, "Influences of Dietary Soy Isoflavones on Metabolism but not Nociception and Stress Hormone Responses in Ovariectomized Female Rats," *Reproductive Biology and Endocrinology* 3 (October 26, 2005):58.

M. B. Zimmermann and J. Köhrle, "The Impact of Iron and Selenium Deficiencies on Iodine and Thyroid Metabolism: Biochemistry and Relevance to Public Health," *Thyroid* 12, no. 10 (October 2002):867–878.

M. G. Gareau, et al., "Probiotic Treatment of Rat Pups Normalizes Corticosterone Release and Ameliorates Colonic Dysfunction Induced by Maternal Separation," *Gut* 56, no. 11 (November 2007):1522–1528.

S. T. Valtysdóttir, L. Wide, and R. Hällgren, "Low Serum Dehydroepiandrosterone Sulfate in Women with Primary Sjögren's Syndrome as an Isolated Sign of Impaired HPA Axis Function," *Journal of Rheumatology* 28, no. 6 (June 2001):1259–1265.

Y. Ishizuki, et al., "The Effects on the Thyroid Gland of Soybeans Administered Experimentally in Healthy Subjects," *Nippon Naibunpi Gakkai Zasshi* 67, no. 5 (May 20, 1991):622–629.

S. D. Johnston, M. Smye, and R. P. Watson, "Intestinal Permeability Tests in Coeliac Disease," *Lancet* 359, no. 9314 (April 13, 2002):1352.

M. E. Sanders and T. R. Klaenhammer, "The Scientific Basis of Lactobacillus Acidophilus NCFM Functionality as a Probiotic," *Journal of Dairy Science* 84, no. 2 (February 2001):319–331.

C. N. Gillis, "Panax Ginseng Pharmacology: A Nitric Oxide Link?" *Biochemical Pharmacology* 54, no. 1 (July 1, 1997):1–8.

A. Grandhi, A. M. Mujumdar, and B. Patwardhan, "A Comparative Pharmacological Investigation of Ashwagandha and Ginseng," *Journal of Ethnopharmacology* 44, no. 3 (December 1994):131–135.

V. Darbinyan, et al., "Rhodiola Rosea in Stress Induced Fatigue—a Double Blind Cross-over Study of a Standardized Extract SHR-5 with a Repeated Low-Dose Regimen on the Mental Performance of Healthy Physicians during Night Duty," *Phytomedicine* 7, no. 5 (October 2000):365–371.

J. S. Zhu, G. M. Halpern, and K. Jones, "The Scientific Rediscovery of an Ancient Chinese Herbal Medicine: Cordyceps Sinensis: Part I," *Journal of Alternative and Complementary Medicine* 4, no. 3 (Fall 1998):289–303.

S. K. Bhattacharya and A.V. Muruganandam, "Adaptogenic Activity of Withania Somnifera: An Experimental Study Using a Rat Model of Chronic Stress," *Pharmacology, Biochemistry and Behavior* 75, no. 3 (June 2003):547–555.

R. Valentino, et al., "Unusual Association of Thyroiditis, Addison's Disease, Ovarian Failure and Celiac Disease in a Young Woman," *Journal of Endocrinological Investigation* 22, no. 5 (May 1999):390–394.

D. F. Neri, et al., "The Effects of Tyrosine on Cognitive Performance during Extended Wakefulness," *Aviation, Space, and Environmental Medicine* 66, no. 4 (April 1995):313–319.

Chapter 7

E. Van Cauter and K. Spiegel, "Sleep as a Mediator of the Relationship between Socioeconomic Status and Health: A Hypothesis," *Annals of the New York Academy of Sciences* 896 (1999):254–261.

A. Tsatsoulis and S. Fountoulakis, "The Protective Role of Exercise on Stress System Dysregulation and Comorbidites," *Annals of the New York Academy of Sciences* 1083 (November 2006):196–213.

"Management of Insomnia: A Place for Traditional Herbal Remedies," *Prescrire International* 14, no. 77 (June 2005):104–107.

L. E. Carlson and S. N. Garland, "Impact of Mindfulness-Based Stress Reduction (MBSR) on Sleep, Mood, Stress and Fatigue Symptoms in Cancer Outpatients," *International Journal of Behavioral Medicine* 12, no. 4 (2005):278–285.

D. W. Spence, et al., "Acupuncture Increases Nocturnal Melatonin Secretion and Reduces Insomnia and Anxiety: A Preliminary Report," *Journal of Neuropsychiatry and Clinical Neurosciences* 16, no. 1 (Winter 2004):19–28.

S. C. Segerstrom, et al., "Optimism Is Associated with Mood, Coping, and Immune Change in Response to Stress," *Journal of Personality and Social Psychology* 74, no. 6 (June 1998):1646–1655.

T. M. Buckley and A. F. Schatzberg, "A Pilot Study of the Phase Angle between Cortisol and Melatonin in Major Depression—a Potential Biomarker?" *Journal of Psychiatric Research* 44, no. 2 (January 2010):69–74.

Chapter 8

J. M. Turner-Cobb, "Psychological and Stress Hormone Correlates in Early Life: A Key to HPA-Axis Dysregulation and Normalisation," *Stress* 8, no. 1 (March 2005):47–57.

O. T. Wolf and B. M. Kudielka, "Stress, Health and Ageing: A Focus on Postmenopausal Women," *Menopause International* 14, no. 3 (September 2008):129–133.

F. Van Den Eede and G. Moorkens, "HPA-Axis Dysfunction in Chronic Fatigue Syndrome: Clinical Implications," *Psychosomatics* 49, no. 5 (September–October 2008):450.

R. S. Lazarus, "Emotions and Interpersonal Relationships: Toward a Person-Centered Conceptualization of Emotions and Coping," *Journal of Personality* 74, no. 1 (February 2006):9–46.

INDEX

General Index

30-Day Adrenal-Friendly Eating Plan Index

ACKNOWLEDGMENTS

I gratefully acknowledge those men and women who have helped me to become all that I am. Without your support, the road would have been far more difficult.

To the wonderful staff at Women to Women who carry the torch on a daily basis. To Carrie, Cate, and Marcy for putting all that we learn into action and for availing so many women the information that is changing their lives.

To Sue, whose calm attitude and amazing work ethic help me immensely and make the chaos become calmer.

To my advocate Jenny, who always has that remarkable insight to help me move forward, and to the wonderful group of people whom I often see on Mondays who keep me clearer.

To Stephanie, who believed in me from the very beginning, and to Janis who helped put the deal together.

To Rachel, whose wonderful words pulled the information together in a seamless way. The book wouldn't be the same without you—you are a genius.

To Frank, the wonderful physician extraodinaire, who has over the years continued to inspire me and continues to be an incredible support.

To Joann, who has been at my side for all these years making sure that the cut worked well in spite of weather and much travel.

To Robert, who keeps my body in great shape and takes the time to assure all is well. A special thanks to Frank and all those at IMT: you always have the answer that facilitates my healing and that reminds me that I do believe in miracles.

To my community of women that supports me and urges me to push beyond what I think is possible: Jane and Laurie.

To Sally, your clear perspective and support have inspired me on a daily basis.

To Linda, for all the wonderful advice about the book and looking forward to the future with your amazing skills.

To Julie, the woman who traverses the uncharted terrain with me, no questions asked. Your support has been greatly appreciated.

To Hay House: Louise Hay, Reid Tracy, Margarete Nielsen, Donna Abate, Laura Koch, and Nancy Levin. Working with you all has taught me that work is joyful and inspiring. To all the people who support the radio show with such gracious ease. Thank you.

To Chris for being the trailblazer that you are. To the initial group that started Women to Women: Chris, Annie, and Ellen. Thank you for believing in our mission.

To Patty Gift, you are truly the best.

To Concordia, for your support with all the wonderful new endeavors we do together.

To Dr. Jeff Bland for reminding me to bridge the gap between the scientific world and the alternative world. To other functional medical practitioners who continue to hold us all accountable in reaching for the best in health-care delivery and service.

To Donna for all your tireless hours of work and recipe developing that created the wonderful food options that we have. I am so grateful for your creative mind and constant inspiration and support.

To my father, who has taught me to pursue the answers and urged me to have a voice.

To Ralph for all your loving support, and to Evan, who never forgets to ask how things are going.

To Joseph for holding down the fort for all these years, and to my wonderful children who keep me on my toes, allowing me to strive to be that much better. You are daily examples of living in balance, understanding that the body is a voice, and that you are what you believe.

To Katya, you continue to amaze me with your tremendous sense of purpose and support. Thank you.

To Micah, your spirit and way of being in the world has much to teach all of us and has been a great teacher for me.

To Josh, the wise young man who is beginning to change the world in his own way, thank you for being you.

ABOUT THE AUTHOR

As co-founder and owner of the world-renowned Women to Women clinic, **Marcelle Pick** has over 25 years of experience working with patients and has worked to change the way in which women's health care is delivered.

In her practice, Marcelle undertakes an integrative approach that not only treats illness, but also educates women to make choices that will help them reach optimal wellness and prevent disease.

Marcelle earned a B.S. in Nursing from the University of New Hampshire, a B.A. in Psychology from the University of New Hampshire, and an M.S. in Nursing from Boston College–Harvard Medical School. She is certified as an OB/GYN nurse-practitioner and a pediatric nurse-practitioner; and is a member of the American Nurses Association, American Academy of Nurse Practitioners, and the American Holistic Nurses Association.

Marcelle has served as medical advisor to *Healthy Living* magazine, lectured on a variety of topics, including "Alternative Strategies to Healing" and "Body Image," and appears regularly in the media discussing women's health. In April 2009 Marcelle's first book, *The Core Balance Diet*, was published by Hay House. She hosts her own radio show, "Core Balance for Women's Health," on Hay House Radio.

Hay House Titles of Related Interest

YOU CAN HEAL YOUR LIFE, the movie, starring Louise L. Hay & Friends
(available as a 1-DVD program and an expanded 2-DVD set)
Watch the trailer at: **www.LouiseHayMovie.com**

THE SHIFT, the movie,
starring Dr. Wayne W. Dyer
(available as a 1-DVD program and an expanded 2-DVD set)
Watch the trailer at: **www.DyerMovie.com**

○ ○ ○

THE ART OF EXTREME SELF-CARE: Transform Your Life One Month at a Time,
by Cheryl Richardson

CALM: A Proven Four-Step Process Designed Specifically for Women Who Worry,
by Denise Marek

FRIED: Why You Burn Out and How to Revive, by Joan Borysenko, Ph.D.

INNER PEACE FOR BUSY WOMEN: Balancing Work, Family, and Your Inner Life,
by Joan Borysenko, Ph.D.

THE SECRET PLEASURES OF MENOPAUSE, by Christiane Northrup, M.D.

All of the above are available at your local bookstore,
or may be ordered by contacting Hay House (see next page).

We hope you enjoyed this Hay House book. If you'd
like to receive our online catalog featuring additional
information on Hay House books and products,
or if you'd like to find out more about the
Hay Foundation, please contact:

Hay House, Inc., P.O. Box 5100, Carlsbad, CA 92018-5100
(760) 431-7695 or (800) 654-5126
(760) 431-6948 (fax) or (800) 650-5115 (fax)
www.hayhouse.com® • www.hayfoundation.org

Published and distributed in Australia by: Hay House Australia Pty. Ltd., 18/36 Ralph St.,
Alexandria NSW 2015 • *Phone:* 612-9669-4299 • *Fax:* 612-9669-4144 • www.hayhouse.com.au

Published and distributed in the United Kingdom by: Hay House UK, Ltd., 292B Kensal Rd.,
London W10 5BE • *Phone:* 44-20-8962-1230 • *Fax:* 44-20-8962-1239 • www.hayhouse.co.uk

Published and distributed in the Republic of South Africa by: Hay House SA (Pty), Ltd.,
P.O. Box 990, Witkoppen 2068 • *Phone/Fax:* 27-11-467-8904 • www.hayhouse.co.za

Published in India by: Hay House Publishers India, Muskaan Complex, Plot No. 3, B-2, Vasant
Kunj, New Delhi 110 070 • *Phone:* 91-11-4176-1620 • *Fax:* 91-11-4176-1630 • www.hayhouse.co.in

Distributed in Canada by: Raincoast, 9050 Shaughnessy St., Vancouver, B.C. V6P 6E5
Phone: (604) 323-7100 • *Fax:* (604) 323-2600 • www.raincoast.com

Take Your Soul on a Vacation

Visit **www.HealYourLife.com®** to regroup, recharge,
and reconnect with your own magnificence.
Featuring blogs, mind-body-spirit news, and
life-changing wisdom from Louise Hay and friends.

Visit **www.HealYourLife.com** today!

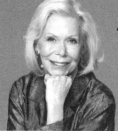